MW00711135

What People Are Saying About "Option Ocean"

"I'm so grateful for this book! I love the honesty and the vulnerability in people telling their stories. The realness of it makes me feel less alone in the ugly things I tell myself sometimes. Thank you for this book and pointing everything back to the One who loves us the most!"

—Jen Snyder

"Kind, inspirational, honest, direct, helpful and very hopeful to ANY young person, or really ANYONE, there is no age limit....good is good. Love it!"

—Maria Luisa Castillo

"This is such an inspiring devotional! All of the personal applications are easy to do, but require you to quiet your heart and listen to yourself!! I found the personal application extremely helpful!"

—April Briggs

"Today's young adults face more options than ever before - a tidal wave that threatens to swamp them once they leave the safe harbor of home. As the mother of two teenage boys, my hope is to equip my sons not just survive the rough seas of life but to chart a course to the joy-filled life God created them to lead.

Option Ocean – Navigating the Sea of Possibility brings together a diverse group of men and women who have successfully weathered perilous storms in their own lives with God's help. Whether your graduates are artistic, athletic, scholarly, or entrepreneurial, these stories will inspire them to pursue their true passions and persevere through the headwinds of adulthood."

—Karen J. Grunst

Option Ocean
Navigating the
Sea of Possibility

Compiled by Kristi Bridges

Book 2 in the 1 Month Wiser Series

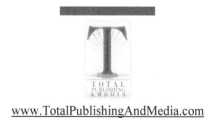

www.TotalPublishingAndMedia.com

ISBN 978-1-63302-121-1

Contents

Week 4: Your Sea Legs are Getting Stronger.

Week 5: Enjoy the Journey!

Introduction

On Labor Day, Tulsa hosts a raft race. People spend weeks building rafts from airplane parts, prom floats, ice chests—and once in a while, actual rafts. Some of those strange parts should never float, but when a clever engineer puts them together, they carry wildly happy crews down the river at high speed.

Over the next 31 days, a few incredible people will help you get to know the Engineer. You may be standing on the shores of possibility, wondering what to do with the parts you've been given. You might have launched out but found yourself floating, your sails limp or leaning precariously. Your Creator wants to work side by side with you to build a life you'd never imagine, using gifts you might think are flaws.

If I were on a raft-building crew, I'd want to know some basics about water and staying on top of it. For example, if you don't caulk your screws, water will fill the raft. Here are some basics for hearing an invisible God in an intrusive world:

- Each day, when you begin your devotional time, pray first. My 90-year-old grandpa Burl has read the Bible every day for 70 years, along with devotions and commentaries. Scripture still helps him. God regularly uses Grandpa's readings to bring him insight and direction.

- Read the context around the verses other people share. It's easy to hear a few motivational words and run with them in the wrong direction. Compare versions of the Christian Bible as well. Grandpa, who has read the Bible in Hebrew and Greek, says the English Standard Version is a pretty reliable translation. However, he and

I both read other versions to get a clear picture and absorb the meaning of what God is showing us.

- As you go through the day, keep your eyes and ears open for God's work around you and ways you can join in.

In this book, you'll meet an award-winning body builder, an artist who doesn't need a day job, and a podcaster who moved across the world for love, years after a map pin foretold it. You'll meet others too, each with stories of what can happen when we let God navigate. As you end each day's devotion, pray with us, and then respond to the journal prompt. We'll end with an action you can take that same day or week. You don't want to simply read about living, right? Where will you go in the Option Ocean?

Week 1: Where Are You Going?

Day 1: Who are you? Ask the I AM.

by Kristi Bridges

Exodus 3 NLT

[11] But Moses protested to God, "Who am I to appear before Pharaoh? Who am I to lead the people of Israel out of Egypt?"

[12] God answered, "I will be with you. And this is your sign that I am the one who has sent you: When you have brought the people out of Egypt, you will worship God at this very mountain."

[13] But Moses protested, "If I go to the people of Israel and tell them, 'The God of your ancestors has sent me to you,' they will ask me, 'What is his name?' Then what should I tell them?"

[14] God replied to Moses, "I AM who I AM. Say this to the people of Israel: I AM has sent me to you."

When my friend moved to Fayetteville for law school, we got our first tattoos in one another's towns.

Lesson learned: Don't get a tattoo in a place you can't reach. My husband doesn't like tattoos. He growled when I came home from Fayetteville, humbly asking him to apply Redemption® aftercare cream to my shoulder blade every night for a week. He took care of me anyway. He's pretty patient.

My friend and I began many adventures at the Blue Rose on Riverside, so we each began with a rose. When I presented the idea to the artist in Fayetteville, I asked him to add a butterfly to symbolize our perpetual state of development. We're different in many ways, but we get a thrill from taking on new challenges. We'll burst out of our cocoons, stretching our wings in delight, then weave new silks from which to evolve once more.

I wasn't always a butterfly. When I was fifteen, my dad called me a chameleon. I told him he was wrong; I was just multi-faceted. Dad was right. I adjusted myself continuously to be whatever the person in front of me seemed to want. If you've ever been around someone who's incessantly shifting to fit you, you know it's very uncomfortable.

I developed this habit as a way to survive. Between first and twelfth grade, I went to eight schools and lived in four households, three of which held extremely volatile step-parents. My natural personality is big. I laugh loudly and sing. I have opinions and voice them. I'm constantly in motion, and I can be a little overwhelming. In many situations, being myself got me in trouble, so being a chameleon seemed like a good defense.

I didn't understand what Dad was telling me, so I kept it up until one day I did real damage. At fifteen, I nearly broke up a marriage. Curled up under my desk in a quilt made from my baby clothes, I contemplated running away. I felt I was a disaster who could do nothing right.

I didn't run. God got my attention and restored me. Repeatedly. Eventually, I learned to let Him lead.

It turns out my tendency to look for ways to connect with people is a gift. I just wasn't using it properly. As a writer, performer, teacher, and friend—even as a customer service representative—I understood where people were coming from and communicated in ways they'd understand. Now that I know who I am, I stay true to myself. This makes others feel comfortable enough to trust me. My gift, developed in sync with its Engineer, has made an impact.

Exodus 2:11-17 tells us that as a young man, Moses dreamed of being a hero but made a mess of things. He killed someone while trying to break up a fight and ended up a fugitive. Decades later in Exodus 3, God told him the time had come: "Tell Pharaoh to let My people go." But because of his previous failure and the years which had passed, Moses felt unqualified.

When God wouldn't accept excuses, Moses asked, "What's Your name, so I can tell him who sent me?"

"I AM," God replied in Exodus 3:14. God answered more than Moses's question. Like many of us, Moses didn't grasp his own identity. He found out who he was when he met the I AM.

Pray.

Lord, I'm curious. Sometimes I feel like I could conquer the world, but other times I feel wrong in so many ways. I recognize that my feelings fluctuate, so I'm going to trust what You say about me. I'd like to know You better and discover myself in the process. Please show me the gifts You've placed in me and guide me as I learn to use them. Thanks, God!

In Jesus's Name, amen.

Think.

Some people make us want to change for the better. Other people convince us to reduce ourselves in an effort to please them. What do you do to nurture positive relationships and protect yourself from people who drag you down?

Act.

This week, observe yourself. When do you feel smart, strong, creative, or compassionate? Ask God to help you use your gifts the way they're intended.

Day 2: Kryptonite

by Kristi Bridges

Proverbs 4 NLT

[1]My children, listen when your father corrects you. Pay attention and learn good judgment, for I am giving you good guidance. Don't turn away from my instructions…[7]Getting wisdom is the wisest thing you can do! And whatever else you do, develop good judgment. [8]If you prize wisdom, she will make you great. Embrace her, and she will honor you…[12]When you walk, you won't be held back; when you run, you won't stumble…[20]My child, pay attention to what I say. Listen carefully to my words. [21]Don't lose sight of them. Let them penetrate deep into your heart, [22]for they bring life to those who find them, and healing to their whole body. [23]Guard your heart above all else, for it determines the course of your life.

When I was four, I floated tummy-down on my dad's hands as he held me up. I was Supergirl! Dad was my Superman for years. I only saw him a couple weeks every summer, but he was strong and good-looking and smart. He knew all the tough-guy lines from *Die Hard* and *Tombstone*. He built fast cars, fast boats, and fast motorcycles, and he loved me. Being loved by a superhero makes a girl feel special.

When I was ten, I read the story of Solomon and asked God for wisdom. I was discovering superheroes don't always make wise choices. Dad got married a lot. When I was thirteen, he revealed his cocaine addiction. He had been through rehab and was clean at the time, but I began to see him as more of an authoritative big brother than a superhero. This wasn't bad. At some point, we must all recognize our parents as people who are experiencing life alongside us. This perspective shifts us from being needy little takers to being partners and fellow travelers.

Dad struggled with coke for years, finally putting down the needle when his kidneys and heart were completely destroyed. After that, he nearly died at least twice a year for ten years. By the time he passed away, I was exhausted. I'd watched him struggle and seen my grandparents worn out. I was angry. I was close to my grandpa and began writing a book of Grandpa's stories, but I was blocked when it came time to write about Dad. I felt like there was no redemption in his story. His suffering was the result of his decisions. All his stories seemed to start with bad decisions and end in tragedy.

Even my good memories of him were splattered in the graffiti of those last years. It took a while for me to scrape it off, but I couldn't finish Grandpa's book without including the second-most important person in his life. Grandma gave me a picture of Dad at two, leaning over the engine of a car. I found a note from a junior high teacher complimenting a drama performance he did. We laughed about how many layers of white it took to cover the giant *Dark Side of the Moon* triangle he'd painted on his living room wall, and I thought of the times we'd sit in the dark listening to music together.

My music has its roots in Dad. I was into mindless pop in ninth grade, and he taught me to respect thought-provoking lyrics and skillful musicians. Mistakes were only part of his story. He'd left each of us kids wiser and more thoughtful.

For Grandpa's last birthday, I gave him the book, including lessons from Dad and a goofy picture of him in a fishing hat and a big, chinny grin.

When I wrote *Wisdom – Better than Wishing*, a 31-day devotional based on the book of Proverbs, I realized just how much Dad had influenced me. When I was twenty-five, I wanted to write books and not just songs, but I felt unready, like my wisdom needed to grow a bit. Long, transparent talks with Dad about relationships and psychology had given me perspective on why we do the things we do. I understood the way minuscule, momentary decisions impact our future. I'm still driven to help people think before they act. I couldn't have written the book without him. Dad's memories and God's wisdom continue to guide my whole business, as I help others build strong relationships, good mental health, and financial wellness.

Is there someone in your life whose flaws frustrate you? Maybe you think they have nothing to teach you. When we embrace wisdom, we learn from everyone God puts in our lives. When we offer love and respect instead of criticism, others learn from us also. My dad made mistakes, but I'd be wrong if I let his errors override the important lessons he taught me.

Even if you have a real hero in your life, make sure to use good judgment. Align your mind with the wisdom of your Creator. Sometimes our heroes get things wrong. I adored my grandpa Fred, but he was raised in a culture of racism. He taught me how to handle money, but I challenged his generalizations about people. We are responsible to check everything against the word of God. Proverbs 4:23 NLT says, "Guard your heart above all else, for it determines the course of your life."

Pray.

Lord, thank You for placing the right people in my life. Give me patience and wisdom as I interact with them. Help me to guard my heart and treat them with respect, even when it's tough. I know You're building skills and understanding that will help me for years to come.

Think.

Think of someone you're having a hard time respecting lately. Thank God for showing you what not to do, then pray for that person. Ask God to fill your heart with love instead of judgment.

Act.

Write down the names of three people who are wise, godly, kind, and successful. Schedule time to spend with each of them this month. Think of a question to ask them and journal about the conversation later.

Day 3: Zone of Genius

by Kristi Bridges

1 Peter 4:10 NIV

Each of you should use whatever gift you have received to serve others, as faithful stewards of God's grace in its various forms.

At work the other day, while my students studied for their licensing exam, I began searching online for art to use in a training piece. I found myself engrossed in optical illusion paintings by Oleg Shuplyak.

I dig optical illusions. From up close, you might see a guy playing guitar, but from across the room, the branch above him becomes a hairline and the guitar becomes some dude's nose. When Oleg was in college, I bet he had a guitar-playing roommate who snored. In any case, his art is impressive. He didn't use some photo app. It took real planning to accomplish these paintings.

From a distance, the life you want to live may look much different than the life you're living now. Up close, your current situation reveals clues you can follow to your best life. In *The Big Leap[1]*, author and therapist Gay Hendricks describes these as road signs to your Zone of Genius. In the Zone of Genius, your life and the lives of others are improved as you use your gifts.

---

[1] Gay Hendricks, *The Big Leap: Conquer Your Hidden Fear and Take Life to the Next Level* (New York: HarperCollins Publishers: 2010*)*.

Zone Check 1.   When you lose yourself for hours in a project or activity, what are you doing?

Zone Check 2.   Which challenges make you feel great about yourself and your impact on the world?

Zone Check 3.   When people show you appreciation, how have you added value to their lives?

Some people know exactly what career they want and focus their whole lives around it. Others have to experiment to find the Zone. They may feel left out because they don't feel a "calling" to anything specific. That's perfectly okay.

There are millions of jobs out there, and they don't all carry fancy titles or giant salaries or public recognition. Every church needs both a pastor and a janitor. Every business needs a CEO and a receptionist. Every celebrity needs an agent. Instead of focusing on money, fame, or importance, hunt for clues about your Zone of Genius. That's where you'll be happiest and most productive. When you're using the gifts God has given you in ways which bring value to others, you'll have everything you need and plenty to share. God will always support His work.

Job 42:2 NIV

I know that you can do all things;
no purpose of yours can be thwarted.

Psalm 115 ESV

¹Not to us, O LORD, not to us, but to your name give glory, for the sake of your steadfast love and your faithfulness! ² Why should the nations say, "Where is their God?" ³ Our God is in the heavens; he does all that he pleases.

Zone Check 4.   If what you're doing is difficult, does it give you a sense of accomplishment? When you're good at it, will you want to keep doing it?

As a customer service representative, I didn't enjoy sitting in one spot for hours at a time. However, hearing my callers' stories made the day fly by. I felt valuable when I could help them understand difficult concepts. When I calmed down an angry caller, I felt like a gold medalist. I developed skills and confidence which improved my personal relationships and creative projects. *Genius clues: I like stories and teaching. I am capable with difficult people.*

I love home remodeling shows. Chip and Joanna Gaines do things I'd never expect, and they add personal creative touches to every home. It gets me excited, so I took a home remodeling class with my husband. I could bounce a nail across the room so fast it would poke a hole in the wall, but I had a hard time sinking the nail into the board I was holding. The circular saw was über fun, and a little practice could improve my hammering skills. Still, I could tell this was not a job I'd want. *Genius clue: Great marriage memory, but a career in carpentry is not for me.*

Zone Check 5.   Does what you're doing contribute to your goals, relationships, or preferred lifestyle? Does it reflect godly values and help others?

As a writer, I'm always astonished by how much time I spend doing things that aren't writing. I do interviews and videos, create promotional art, and network. I also hang out with my husband and friends. Occasionally, I clean house. I have to be intentional about how much time I allot to each activity, so I have healthy relationships and finished books.

My most important time is spent reading the Bible and praying each morning. In business, we have calibration meetings. In these meetings, we align our understanding and activities to the boss's plans. God wants a vibrant relationship with us that goes far beyond that of boss and employee, but calibration time is still extremely important. Without it, I could easily veer from the Lord's best for me. I could find my time sucked away and accomplish nothing. By spending time with Him in the morning, I begin a conversation that will last all day: *Lord, help me to reflect the fruits of the Spirit. Guard my time. Show me what You're doing, so I can join in.*

Pray.

Thank You, Lord, for the gifts and talents You've given me. Thank You for opportunities to try new things and develop useful skills and insight. What would You like to show me today?

Think.

Draw a line down the middle of a piece of paper. Break down what you've done in the past day, week, or month. In the first column, list activities which brought you enjoyment or a sense of accomplishment. In the second column, list activities you would not want to do on a regular basis.

For each activity in the first column, do a Zone Check using these three questions:

1. When you get really good at this, will you want to keep doing it?
2. Does this contribute to your goals, relationships, or preferred lifestyle?
3. Does it reflect godly values and help others?

Act.

In this stage of your work life, you'll probably have to do quite a few tasks which aren't in your Zone of Genius. Do them to the best of your ability because integrity matters. Look for ways you can spend the majority of your time blessing others in ways that light you up.

Day 4: Set Your Compass

by Richard Staley, PhD.

I Corinthians 13:11 NKJV

When I was a child, I spoke as a child, I understood as a child, I thought as a child; but when I became a man, I put away childish things.

When I was a freshman in high school, I wrote a paper on what I wanted to do after high school and college. I chose the career of architecture. I didn't really know much about it, but I had a good friend who said that's what he wanted to do. I wasn't good at math, so that didn't work out too well. I floundered, exploring several other careers that didn't seem to fit either. My first college degree was in business administration. That's a great degree, and I learned a lot from that path of study, but it was not my thing. After a lot of frustration and prayer, I realized I had a gift for teaching. I went back to college, got three more degrees, and ended up teaching, being an administrator, and finally serving as a university professor. There is a note of humor in all this. In my late teens and young adult years, I adamantly said the one thing I would never be was a teacher, particularly a high school teacher. My first teaching position was with students in junior high and high school. Be careful what you say; you may have to eat your words.

Becoming a man or woman is not arriving at a final point. Rather, it is a continuous process. Learning and growing is a lifelong activity. If we quit, we stop moving forward and start moving backward.

In your teen and early adult years, you've most likely heard, "You can be anything you want to." That is a popular statement, but for the child of God, it is not exactly true. Consider Jeremiah 1:4-5 NKJV: "⁴ Then the word of the Lord came to me saying: ⁵ Before I formed you in the womb I knew you; before you were born I sanctified you; I ordained you a prophet to the nations."

This verse applies to every born-again child of God. He had a plan for your life before you were born. This wasn't just for Jeremiah the prophet; it is for everyone. You may not be called by God into full-time ministry, but He called you to fulfill a particular purpose. Dissatisfaction, frustration, and a multitude of other issues come from doing what you want to do or what others have said you should do, instead of what God wants you to do.

The question becomes, "How do I know what God wants me to do with my life?" Here are some steps you can take to answer that question:

1. Put the Word of God first, every day.

2. Make prayer part of your daily routine.

3. Listen for the Holy Spirit to speak to you. He usually speaks, so you hear a still, small voice with your spirit, not with your physical ears.

4. Whatever He says to you, do it.

You might ask, "Why are these things important?" Let's find out.

Putting the Word of God first will enable you to really know God. Psalm 138:2 NKJV says, "I will worship toward Your holy temple, and praise Your name, for Your lovingkindness and Your truth; for You have magnified Your word above all Your name." God has some very impressive names, but this verse says He has magnified His word above His name. You will find out that He is faithful; He is love; His mercy endures forever, and He cares about you.

Making prayer part of your daily routine gives you an opportunity to have a relationship with the Most High. Prayer is not just you talking and telling God what you want and need. It is communication. For communication to occur, both individuals have to take part in the conversation. You should not only talk; you should listen.

Listening for God to speak is sometimes difficult for people, and some folks say things like, "God never speaks to me." But that is contrary to what God's word says. John 10:4 NKJV says, "And when He brings out His own sheep, He goes before them; and the sheep follow Him, for they know His voice." God is always speaking.

James 1:22 NKJV says, "But be doers of the word, and not hearers only, deceiving yourselves." John 2:5 NKJV says, "His mother said to the servants, 'Whatever He says to you, do it.'" When we hear God speaking through His word or by the voice of the Holy Spirit, we must act. If we don't, we are disobeying and deceiving ourselves into thinking something other than what God is saying.

Romans 12:1-2 NKJV tells us we will be transformed as we put God first in our lives. "[1] I beseech you therefore, brethren, by the mercies of God, that you present your bodies a living sacrifice, holy, acceptable to God, which is your reasonable service. [2] And do not be conformed to this world, but be transformed by the renewing of your mind, that you may prove what is that good and acceptable and perfect will of God." God's perfect will is better than any other path you might try.

I'm praying for you. Would you like to pray with me?

Pray.

Father, in the name of Jesus I come before You and present myself. I ask for Your help in setting my priorities in order. I will put Your word first, listen and hear Your voice, and do what I hear You say. I know You have a plan for my life, and I desire to be in Your perfect will. Thank You for guiding me by your Holy Spirit. In Jesus's name, Amen.

Think.

How will you rearrange your daily activities so you can discover what God's plan is for your life?

Act.

What will you do differently, starting tomorrow morning?

Day 5: Picked up on a Wave

by Rip Kastaris

Ephesians 2:10 NLT

For we are God's masterpiece. He has created us anew in Christ Jesus, so we can do the good things he planned for us long ago.

I don't know if anybody really chooses art. You get picked up in it like you get picked up in a wave when you're playing on the beach in shallow water. For me, it started in kindergarten. We were painting, but there was no white. My teacher was surprised when I complained. She said, "Euripides, you have six other colors. Why don't you paint with what you have?"

"I can't mix the lighter colors unless I have the white."

Later, while the other kids napped, she came to me and said, "Rip, you don't have to sleep." That's when I realized art could get me out of all kinds of stuff. We went into a supply room and she said, "Because you asked for the white, you can help me mix up this white tempera paint."

In second grade, my art was taken as samples for the next class. In fourth grade, I had a very ambitious teacher. She was making a slide show of a Brazilian story called "The Red Shoes," and she was on a deadline. If you were good at illustration, you didn't have to do your math work.

I was very fortunate to have high school art teachers who saw promise. When I was sixteen, they got me into a program at Washington University in St. Louis. It's one of the best art schools in the country. Through the program, I spent my last two years of high school at the university drawing directly from a model and seeing work being done by undergraduate and graduate students. I was offered a scholarship to Parsons School of Design in New York, but I stayed in St. Louis at Washington University.

It was a marvelous education in the arts, but also in other things. I never checked the levels of my classes. We had to take core courses such as history and biology, so I'd ask upperclassmen, "What got under your skin?" I realized if I took classes that were interesting- things I could get passionate about- I could pass no matter what level it was.

Two years before I graduated, I was offered a job. It happened while I was volunteering. My roommate's sister was working on her master's degree in social work. She created an agency called Kids in the Middle. It served kids whose parents were divorcing, helping them to not feel guilty about what was happening with their parents and not to be used as pawns in their parents' battle. I did pen and ink illustrations for the project with someone who owned an ad agency. He liked my work and told me when I graduated, I had a place.

Everything is designed—the pen you use, the shirt you wear. It's much easier to get a job in design than a job in illustration, so in spite of wanting to do illustration, it made sense to take the design job he offered. While starting in design, I took freelance jobs as an illustrator. I was the king of the all-nighter, and one day my boss came in and said, "You've been up all night. What are you going to be able to do for me today?"

I said, "I can do this. I can handle it."

He said, "But really, Rip, what do you want to do with your career and your life?"

I said, "Someday, I really want to be an illustrator." He said, "You can be an illustrator this afternoon." He thought he was funny. I did not, but he did me a favor by letting me go.

My boss and I made a plan where I'd be fired from working full-time but continue as a freelance designer. That year, I made more as a freelancer for him than I would have working full time, and all the while, I added six more clients. I was off to the races doing freelance work for Ralston Purina, Energizer, Anheuser-Busch, Winchester, and other big agencies working between New York and St. Louis. I was so happy.

Art is a different type of intelligence, and it's often pursued by people who don't have another way to express themselves. As a kid, I felt like an outsider, because my name was Euripides rather than Rick or Bill, and my family had moved over from Greece. My way of seeing things was different than other kids. I'm an artist; I solve every problem with art. When my goddaughter was baptized, I made her a Greek Orthodox icon. I didn't know what else to do for her. If I need to make a contribution to my church, I donate art. If I need therapy, I make art. If I need to make a living, I make art. If I need to arrange furniture, I draw it out and use art to make it work properly.

My guidance counselor in high school did not have faith in me, telling me they didn't take people like me at Washington University. Now, when I go back for career day, she has to pin the badge on me. We need to realize that one sentence of discouragement could change a life in the wrong way, but that also means one word of encouragement can bring hope. We need to encourage ourselves and others. We must be able to work past the negative comments of others. Everyone can use their individual God-given gifts to create. Everything we talk about or touch or drive was someone's idea. We are made in the image of our Creator, and we can all be creative. Anyone that is fully functioning and expressing themselves cannot help but create.

Pray.

Creator of heaven and earth, You made us in Your image. I am your living enterprise. Even when I don't feel creative, if I tune into You and examine my life, I can be inspired to find my way. What I see in part can become blessed, abundant, and meaningful in service to others, as I develop, seeing things unfold as whole and divine through You. I will do my part. I will work with faith, but without expectations for immediate results. I will express talents and desires that You, Yourself have created in me. Thank You for giving me life and passion.

Think.

Look back at your life, from elementary school to now. Think about the moments where you felt passionate, curious, or successful. Maybe you even got into trouble, but in those moments can you see a talent or drive God placed in you?

Act.

Talk to God first, then speak to a guidance counselor or career coach about jobs where you can use that talent or drive. Not all guidance counselors are negative. Find mentors, people who are already doing what you love for a living, and risk getting rejected to share what you do for their opinion and advice. They often know about possibilities we haven't discovered. Then find ways to use your talent to help others.

Day 6: Confluence

by Kristi Bridges and Rip Kastaris

Genesis 12 NLT

[1] *The Lord had said to Abram, "Leave your native country, your relatives, and your father's family, and go to the land that I will show you.* [2] *I will make you into a great nation. I will bless you and make you famous, and you will be a blessing to others.* [3] *I will bless those who bless you and curse those who treat you with contempt. All the families on earth will be blessed through you."*

In St. Louis, Missouri, the Mississippi river turns back on itself, flowing northeast for a few miles before coming back and forming a confluence with the Missouri river. From there, the strengthened Mississippi flows toward the Gulf of Mexico. Cities thrive on its banks.

I met Rip Kastaris at a Greek festival in Tulsa. My friend and I had gone for food and culture, but as we rounded a corner, I froze in place. Baklava would have to wait. I couldn't take my eyes off the paintings of Buddy Guy, BB King, Bob Marley, Sting, and musicians I hadn't yet discovered. My ears heard traditional Greek accordion, but my soul felt knee-melting guitar riffs coming from the canvas.

Mingled with the blues were other paintings, Byzantine-era depictions of Mary, Jesus, and the disciples. Their heads were tilted and circled in gold like images I'd seen in my college Humanities class. Rip said hi, and I commented that I'd never seen one artist use such completely disparate styles so well. An hour later, we were still talking when my friend said, "Kristi! Baklava!" We hadn't yet run out of things to talk about. I've been following Rip ever since.

Like the Mississippi, Rip's career has turned back and returned to pick up new partnerships and new ideas. Knowing that, it makes sense that my favorite piece is *Confluence*, a mural he did on Broadway in St. Louis.

I had the pleasure of interviewing him during the *Hope to Hope* conference in March of 2018. He was a few months into a year-long project, painting the inside of St. Josaphat's Ukrainian Catholic Cathedral in Parma, Ohio.

"I had not planned on being an artist who was climbing sixty-five feet in the morning to paint Christ in a dome with a brush that's duct-taped to sticks longer than me. When I was fresh out of college, I told my friends I was glad my parents moved our family from Greece to the US, because if we'd stayed in Greece I'd be stuck doing churches.

"I think we become more of ourselves over time, because after ten years of advertising art, I felt like I was just about half an inch deep. I went back to Greece and toured the churches. As a child, I once looked at a book and commented how beautiful a cathedral was, and they said, 'We came out with that book for our 1600th birthday.' 1600 years! Seeing them in person made me think differently about the images we look at all day. Madonna had hits for a while, but the Madonna and Child have been a hit for thousands of years.

"I was asked to do shows with other Greek artists because of being part of the Orthodox church and that social group. When I did icons, everybody responded, even those who were non-Greeks."

Basing our actions on the response of others has merit. The first rule of successful business is to find out what people need or want. Doing slides for his teacher, volunteering for Kids in the Middle, and taking a design job at an ad agency helped Rip develop understanding and skills which make him versatile and in high demand. Besides paying the bills, it's fun to have variety in your work. Plus, it feels good to be appreciated.

People can box us into a single set of expectations, though. What if Rip had never reached beyond teaching slides or ad design? He wouldn't have been commissioned to paint by both the US and Greek Olympic Committees. As we become experts at one thing, we should keep our minds and skillsets growing. When we try new things just for fun, we discover new passions and ways to express our talents. When we stay alert to what God is doing around us, we can join Him at work and be ready for opportunities He brings us.

"It's a struggle for many, many people," Rip says. "Do I follow my still, small voice or do what's expected of me? We think good people live up to expectations of society, their parents, their spouses, and kids. I think it takes a little insight and a little courage to step out of what's been done. We have to ask ourselves some serious questions to live up to our calling.

"There's tension whenever somebody chooses to go the route of inspiration instead of duty.

"We have to work to go from the people we are to the people God has made us in spirit. We have the blueprint of our Creator. We yearn, but it takes not hitting the snooze button, practicing without witnesses, missing a vacation your friends are taking in order to go from good to great. We're all capable, but we're not all willing. Maybe it's fine to have a normal life, but there is a call to adventure in all stories.

"In today's life when everything is so easy, what people really need is not a faster car or a bigger house, they need experiences where they don't feel like a number in a system that's so large they have no influence. Most people yearn for a connection with their kids and their grandparents and a sense they're working towards something that's going to allow them to make a living but will also leave a legacy.

"Be courageous. Be a little heroic. Realize you're under the same sun as those who've come before you and done great things. You can, too."

Pray.

Lord, I want to be fully alive while I'm living. Help me to focus and develop the talents You've given me. Give me fortitude when I need to stick with something that pays and inspiration when there are new avenues to explore. I trust You to open doors when You know I'm ready to walk through them.

Think.

Have there been times when you've flitted from one thing to another without developing expertise at anything? What can you do right now to develop pro-level skill at one thing you enjoy doing?

Act.

Make time to heighten your skills. You might need to get up earlier, or you might want to participate in a group project where you'll have accountability.

Day 7: A Pin in the Map

by Cyndilu Miller

Daniel 7 NLT

[13] As my vision continued that night, I saw someone like a son of man coming with the clouds of heaven. He approached the Ancient One and was led into his presence. [14] He was given authority, honor, and sovereignty over all the nations of the world, so that people of every race and nation and language would obey him. His rule is eternal—it will never end. His kingdom will never be destroyed.

My friend had a ministry in her garage, and I was with her from the beginning. It became known as the "White Horse Cave," and missionaries from all over the world came to the garage to share what God was doing around the globe. One day, we were standing in her dining room making "God Lists" of places we'd like to go. She had a map of the world on her wall, so we put virtual pins on various countries as we talked. Peru had come to us, so of course we put Peru on the list. My friend wanted to go to India, and I wanted to go to Africa. Then I pointed to a country on the opposite corner of the map. Standing in Vermont I said, "I want to go to New Zealand, but I know I can't go until I'm ready to stay. I know I'm going to want to stay awhile."

I was still in my first marriage, with a man who was challenged to travel to the next state, so I wondered how this could be. A few years later, the marriage ended, and I remembered New Zealand. I was nowhere near ready to go there. I needed to learn who I was and what I liked, to discover my gifts, and heal from years of feeling worthless and being neglected by the person who was supposed to love me. God had given me strength during those years, but now He'd given me freedom.

I focused on my friends from church. They were encouraging and fun, and a couple years after my divorce, they told me about a guy at church. "Robin's from New Zealand, Cyndilu. Isn't that interesting? Maybe you two should get to know each other."

"No way!" I said. Robin was scruffy. I found out later that was because he worked nights and came to church exhausted after his shift. At first glance though, I said, "No, no, no. He's not my type."

I'd talk to my friends about the kind of man I'd like to marry one day, and they'd say, "Well you know, that sounds an awful lot like Robin." They just didn't get it. I didn't want scruffy—I wanted a man who was put together.

Eventually, after a challenge from Robin—another story—I started to talk with him. Within a month, I realized they were right. Nine months later, he asked me to marry him. He is the most wonderful, amazing scruffy man I will ever, ever have the honor and privilege of being married to!

Every relationship we have affects our future relationships. Abusive and neglectful situations in my youth caused me to attract abusers. I never meant to end up in a failed first marriage, but I didn't recognize clues in our chemistry which blended to create an abysmal situation. After taking time to discover myself and learn to relate to healthy people, I was able to recognize the type of man with whom I could create a happy life. Even then, it took work. We had to patiently wade through our learned responses. There were times I treated him as though he was exactly the same as my first husband. He's a completely different person, kind and compassionate. He patiently helped me to see that.

When I landed in New Zealand, I knew I was home. We were able to spend time with his mother while she was alive, and we found a supportive, vibrant church. I've learned a few words. My car has a boot instead of a trunk, and I wear lippy instead of lipstick. Today, I help others uncover their own talents and dream about their futures. It's wild to think God gave me a map pin, years before I arrived, to get me excited about His plan. What hints has God given you? Follow wisdom and trust His timing, and you'll see them come true.

Globe-hopping tip: If you decide to move across the world, sell everything you can easily replace. Don't try to move all your stuff from one country to another. Research prices before you sell, though. If we'd done that, we would have brought Robin's carpentry tools.

Pray.

Thank You Lord for giving us clues to Your plan. Protect and guide me. If I have behaviors or preferences which would land me in destructive relationships, point them out and change my heart. If I react to new people based on those who've hurt me, adjust my reactions. Help me to choose wisely and proceed in patience. I look forward to going everywhere You want to take me. In Jesus's Name.

Think.

Do you have a White Horse Cave—people in your life who enjoy talking about what God has done? When you have a choice between news, chatter, or testimony, why not choose stories that express God's love and power? At www.Guidepost.org and www.christian-faith.com/ you can find stories which will have you eagerly watching for God's work around you.

Act.

Start a conversation among your friends. Ask, "Has God ever given you a hint about your future that isn't happening yet?"

Week 2:Who's at the Helm?

Day 8: Pressure v Power

by Sarah Soon and Kristi Bridges

Ephesians 3 NLT

[16] I pray that from his glorious, unlimited resources he will empower you with inner strength through his Spirit. [17] Then Christ will make his home in your hearts as you trust in him. Your roots will grow down into God's love and keep you strong. [18] And may you have the power to understand, as all God's people should, how wide, how long, how high, and how deep his love is. [19] May you experience the love of Christ, though it is too great to understand fully. Then you will be made complete with all the fullness of life and power that comes from God.

[20] Now all glory to God, who is able, through his mighty power at work within us, to accomplish infinitely more than we might ask or think. [21] Glory to him in the church and in Christ Jesus through all generations forever and ever! Amen.

Today's verses are at the heart of everything we'd like to say to our younger selves, to you, and to every other human on the planet. If there are aliens, we want them to have this hope as well!

Before we began writing this book, we wrote letters to our younger selves. When I read this one, I wished Sarah Soon had been around when I went to college. God's power accomplishes infinitely more than we can imagine.

Dear Sarah,

I know you're about to venture into life, moving away from home to attend ORU and discovering who you are. All at eighteen. Seems like life is moving slow because the day to day grind of working in the summer, packing your stuff, and re-checking if you have everything feels monotonous; yet, fast as moving day draws closer and your checklist grows longer. Rest assured, everything happens in its time.

You want to learn as much as possible, but you feel pressure to perform. You want to obtain all A's like in high school, but the feat seems more daunting at the university level.

Can you withstand all the pressure? Because you're about to step into the future, these steps feel daunting. One misstep might mean a demotion or slammed door to a prestigious law school.

And there's the whole social life issue as well. Of course, you expect to not only date, but find your lifelong mate (didn't intend to rhyme). That almost seems fraught with more danger than the career journey, doesn't it?

Finally, there's God. Where does He play in this journey?

First of all, let me assure you that all the mysteries of your next chapter will culminate in growth. The uncertainty is exactly where God wants you. Yes, it's terrifying, stressful (sorry, you broke out with ache patches), and exciting, all at the same time. Failure seems all but inevitable. Success feels obscure.

But have peace—you only need to take it a day at a time.

Breathe even when plans don't go your way, because you'll have plenty of those days. But it's not about the B's — you'll get two but in PE, not academic courses— because you learn how to learn. You'll not retain as much as you expected, but that's the beauty. It's about learning how to learn, discovering how you can expand your mind and challenge yourself to new frontiers whether in business, humanities, earth science, and well, the new horizon that will shape your life- English. You're having a difficult time swallowing that one, but trust.

I don't want to spoil your journey and faith, but focus on giving your best. Learn, study, and value your professors. Your attitude towards your peers, your professors, and your mentors is invaluable and plays as much a part in your success as your performance factors: grades, standing, and attendance.

Find time to not only have fun but explore opportunities. Don't let money and time stop you. Go on the European Humanities trip and the Grand Canyon hiking trip. Volunteer your time to causes you love — which you will, but make sure it's what you want to do. Open your heart and door to your friends, both male and female. Bond more with your brother wing buddies. Ask them questions and get to know the opposite sex in a safe and comfortable light. You'll need their friendship to navigate through life, trust me.

And realize that the more you ask questions, the greater the growth. Don't take one-on-one time with friends, professors, and peers lightly, but live in the moment. That test will still be waiting for you once you return to your room. Think outside of the box and don't take yourself too seriously. Laugh more, learn beyond the classroom, and ask probing questions.

And about the boyfriend, don't be impatient. Just embrace your singleness, go out with your male friends, and appreciate who they are as men. You won't find a husband at ORU, but make this time invaluable by getting to know how to communicate with the opposite sex, discover what makes them tick, and learn what they want and need as friends.

And your siblings. You'll enjoy getting to know them better. Enjoy every moment with them because you'll value and need their friendship throughout your life.

One last thing, God. This relationship becomes the most important one. You will cling to Him, grow in knowledge of Him, and draw nigh to His love. This will help establish you once you graduate and go off on your own.

So live life to the fullest, trust God, and embrace uncertainty!

Sincerely,
Your older self.

Pray.

Lord, how do I rest in You when there's so much going on? I'm determined to put You first. Would you please teach me how to prioritize, so I can get the truly important things done while getting closer to You day by day? Thank You! I love You so much.

Think.

How do you respond to pressure? Do you stress out or procrastinate? When you ask for help, do you do your part? When you're helping others, do you ignore your own work?

Act.

Write a letter to yourself today, from yourself one year in the future (if you're eighteen, write a letter from your nineteen-year-old self). Pretend this year has already ended and thank yourself for what you did right. Describe your accomplishments and give yourself some encouragement.

Day 9: Your Real Name

by Kristi Bridges

Revelations 2 NLT

[17] *"Anyone with ears to hear must listen to the Spirit and understand what he is saying to the churches. To everyone who is victorious I will give some of the manna that has been hidden away in heaven. And I will give to each one a white stone, and on the stone will be engraved a new name that no one understands except the one who receives it.*

I'm six years old, sitting in a dark hallway with my classmates, trying to stay quiet like the teacher said, but how does a six-year-old stay quiet? I have so much to say! I'm wearing my yellow dress. The boy across the street (who always shoots me down when we pretend we're in Star Wars) says it makes me look like a butterfly. Apparently, yellow butterflies get defective force fields, but wait! Ssh! We're moving! Single-file, we cross the stage, and now it's okay to speak. I speak to the clock in the back of the cafeteria, just like the teacher said. Then we all sing a song, as loud as we can, and it's the best feeling I've felt in all 1,971 days of my life. The part of me I was meant to be is ALIVE!

From that day on, I sing Dorothy's song while on my swing set every afternoon. I'm a bluebird wanting to fly. Who needs a wizard? I only want a Hollywood agent to discover me, as he wanders through the woods in Beulah behind my house, because I think that's where agents go to scout new talent.

At six, I decided I'd run off to Hollywood the moment I graduated. Most kids change dreams periodically, but for me, it wasn't just a career choice. I claimed "actress" as my identity. This was useful, even though I didn't get any more speaking roles for several years. I went to eight schools, and being dramatic gave me confidence and the determination to rise above rejection.

I needed that determination. In sixth grade, a classmate called me names from the other end of the lunch table every day for two weeks. I returned the favor but finally broke and ran to the bathroom crying.

On my thirteenth birthday, I was dressed like Madonna, washing dishes to prepare for my party. My then-stepfather sat at the kitchen table in his usual dark mood, calling me similar names. I'd have traded my fingerless gloves for boxing gloves in an instant. Finally, I lost my temper and mouthed off. He canceled my slumber party.

In the next few years, I got a few roles. My characters were the over-the-top type who died in the first act. Off-stage, I sought a twisted kind of respect by living up to the names I'd been called.

When people label us, we might fight back at first, and then find ourselves defiantly living up to their labels. We can't stop their insults, so we act like they're not so bad. We wear hateful names as badges of honor. It's a survival technique, but God has a better way.

Our Creator is the only One who was with us before we were born and will be with us every place we go. We'll leave the snobs, the users, the bullies behind and keep moving forward in the plans He has for us. He will uncover our true identities, like layers of one Christmas gift wrapped around another, until at last we pull out a white identity stone which truly describes us.

Sound good? What can we do?

No matter how you feel about yourself and even if you've repeated some mistakes, read God's thoughts about you. When Jeremiah 31 was written, He was speaking to Israel, but the Lord gives His heart to every person who loves Him. He's speaking to you through His word today.

Jeremiah 31 NLT

³Long ago the Lord said to Israel: "I have loved you, my people, with an everlasting love. With unfailing love I have drawn you to myself. ⁴I will rebuild you, my virgin Israel. You will again be happy and dance merrily with your tambourines. ⁵Again you will plant your vineyards on the mountains of Samaria and eat from your own gardens there."

God loves you faithfully and wants to restore your innocence so you'll be lighthearted and dancing. He sees you doing something profitable and enjoying the results of your labor.

Pause for a moment and SEE what God sees. Absorb it. God's word is reality.

Now, take a look at these verses. Can you see some of these qualities inside yourself? Can you see some you'd like to strengthen?

Colossians 3:12 NLT

Since God chose you to be the holy people he loves, you must clothe yourselves with tenderhearted mercy, kindness, humility, gentleness, and patience.

1 Corinthians 9 NLT

²⁵All athletes are disciplined in their training. They do it to win a prize that will fade away, but we do it for an eternal prize.

²⁶So I run with purpose in every step. I am not just shadowboxing.

Proverbs 22:1 ESV

A good name is to be chosen rather than great riches, and favor is better than silver or gold.

Pray.

Lord, You've heard the things people have said about me and seen how I've acted unlike the me You created. You know how it feels. People lie about You, too. Thank You for being right here, breathing love and truth and hope into my life. I will contemplate Your vision every day. I will revel in innocence and enjoy the results of the work You give me.

Think.

What do you think your identity stone will say? Write a few sentences describing your talents, special quirks, and godly characteristics.

Act.

Be the person who sincerely points out the good in people. Pray before speaking and don't be overwhelming or gushy, but be the voice which reminds them of their true selves, created by God.

Day 10: PICK Your Life

by Kristi Bridges

Ecclesiastes 11:4 NLT

*Farmers who wait for perfect weather never plant.
If they watch every cloud, they never harvest.*

Proverbs 22:13 NLT

*The lazy person claims, "There's a lion out there! If I go
outside, I might be killed!"*

When I was in eighth grade, I learned about computers on a TRS80. We call it a Trash 80, because even back then, it was outdated. The operating system was DOS, and I learned how to write an astronomy program in BASIC (Beginner's All-purpose Symbolic Instruction Code). I saved it on a 5 ¼ inch floppy disc made of translucent black plastic. The disc had a flimsy plastic cover, because if you touched the floppy, your fingerprints would wreck the program.

What if I had boxed up that floppy disc? What if I'd wrapped it in colorful paper, added a bow, and held onto it for all these years? "I have a gift," I would say, as each year came and went. If I didn't share the gift or let anyone use it, it would become more and more outdated. What if instead, I shared the gift unashamedly and joyfully? That disc held my first programming attempt in eighth grade, so it might not have won an award, but someone might have used it to learn the difference between quasars and black holes. They might have given me feedback, so I could further develop my gift.

Feedback is scary. We hide our gifts sometimes, fearing what others will say. Rick Warren, author of *The Purpose-Filled Life*, warns, "Perfectionism paralyzes potential." Which is better? Going back to the drawing board with feedback and developing Gift 2.0 or watching others accomplish things we only dream about?

Instead of a floppy piece of useless plastic in a pretty box, I could have a string of successes. The StarMap 3D app on my phone was the result of such an evolution. When I point my phone at the sky, this app tells me the names of constellations, stars, and planets. In a few years, it will be replaced by virtual reality, but tonight I'm having fun with it.

What is burning in your heart? Maybe you're contemplating corporate jobs but dreaming of being an artist, singer, speaker, or personal trainer. Go for it! Enter an art show. Perform at an open mic. Join a Toastmasters group. Lead a Bible study, sing in church, hone your skills, and share them wherever God opens doors.

A wise and godly business coach will teach you how to earn a living, even if you must work a "day job" while building your market. God enjoys providing when we do His work. It's the law of generosity. The more we share what He's given us, the more He provides. Then we have more to share.

After keeping my gifts to myself for several years, I said, "I want to write, even if I'm just writing songs in my backyard." I scheduled writing dates with myself. Then I picked a couple of songs to sing a capella at open mic poetry readings. I met musicians, formed bands, and learned a lot about communicating my ideas to instrumentalists. I also gained confidence and skills which resulted in pay raises and promotions at my day job. I didn't make millions in music, but it paid for itself and strengthened the faith of countless people. Plus, I made amazing memories and even better friends.

When I moved into writing books and speaking, I began by going to Toastmasters meetings for practice and connections. Whatever your gift, there's a place to develop it.

When people put all their efforts into building a safe life, they hide their unpolished gifts and often end up feeling trapped. By forty, they want to run away and express themselves. They may wreck relationships, finances, or health and end up awash in regret. Why go that route when you could be responsibly creative now?

PICK your life.

Phrase with Power

Eliminate the following phrases from your vocabulary:

- "I'd love to, but I can't."
- "I wish I could, but I don't have enough time."
- "I can't afford that."

Those phrases reinforce a sense of lack. Lack feeds the temptation to be reckless. You get to choose how you'll spend your money and time, so follow Jesus's advice in Matthew 5:37 NLT: "Just say a simple, 'Yes, I will,' or 'No, I won't.'"

Insist on Your Dream

Make decisions in favor of what means the most to you. You may have to choose between movie night with friends and making a fruit sculpture for the catering business you're starting. Friends are important, but instead of whining about missing the fun, give yourself a high five for following your dream!

Collaborate and Get Wise Counsel

It's easier to stay on track if you're working with someone else. Get good counsel from a business coach and try small, project-based collaborations. This will give you accountability and expand your advertisement. You'll each tell your own set of friends what you're doing, and pretty soon everyone will know. Collaborating on single, small projects gives you the chance to escape when the project is finished. When there's no end in sight, some collaborations result in disappointment, failed commitments. and busted friendships.

Know the Cost

While you're practicing, you might give away your talents, but if you want them to pay one day, track the money and time each project takes. Proverbs 20:25 NIV says, "It is a trap to dedicate something rashly and only later to consider one's vows." When you can calculate your effort and expenses, you'll make reasonable commitments you can keep. In business, reliability is highly valued.

Pray.

Lord, I love You. Thank You for curiosity and the ability to enjoy doing things others might not. Please forgive me for times I've been lazy or procrastinated due to insecurity about the gifts You've given me. I'm ready to put this potential to use. Please show me what steps to take.

Think.

You think differently than any other human being. When something sparks and holds your attention, you take it in directions which might surprise others. "God don't make junk," they say in the South. What have you done or thought of doing, which you would enjoy developing?

Act.

Begin today. Tonight, write down what you did, and the step you'll take tomorrow.

Day 11: Follow Wisdom

by Premadonna Braddick, MA

Proverbs 4 NIV

[5] Get wisdom, get understanding;
do not forget my words or turn away from them.

[6] Do not forsake wisdom, and she will protect you;
love her, and she will watch over you.

[7] The beginning of wisdom is this: Get wisdom.
Though it cost all you have, get understanding.

[8] Cherish her, and she will exalt you; embrace her,
and she will honor you.

[9] She will give you a garland to grace your head
and present you with a glorious crown.

In March of 2013, I had just finished hosting another incredible Girls' Teen Summit. I was exhausted but happy. The Summit is huge, consisting of workshops and panels for junior and high school girls. Speakers pour into the young ladies while simultaneously breaking down the walls they've built. Workshops delve into topics such as bullying, financial literacy, college readiness, sex trafficking, mental illness, drug abuse, health and fitness, domestic violence, career planning, and much more.

Many people ask how I was inspired to put on an event like this. I had a couple of reasons. It saddened me to hear that Oklahoma has the highest female incarceration rate in the nation.[2] I heard the Lord tell me to go get His teen girls, so they wouldn't become sad statistics. The second reason was my personal story. I grew up in the foster care system and aged out because no one wanted to adopt me. Yeah, you can imagine the years of rejection I felt. To top that off, in some of my foster homes, I endured countless incidents of sexual, physical, and verbal abuse. It didn't help to have one of my foster mothers tell me the only reason she took me into her home was to be a playmate for her biological daughter. Now, that was a blow to a little five-year-old who dreamed of a loving family welcoming her!

I was determined to help other girls overcome their circumstances, and news of my Girls' Teen Summit spread throughout Tulsa, Oklahoma. We were invited to use a bigger facility for the next year on a weekend. I had been hosting the Summit during school hours when we were certain to get a lot of girls. I remembered the fun of field trips. What student didn't want a day away from school?

A weekend Summit? I would be responsible for getting the girls there. I panicked, but then thought, "No biggie. I will just talk to Sandy." Sandy is a seasoned conference host who had helped me with the prior two Summits. We helped each other out with a variety of events we hosted for the youth. I came to her office with a big smile and said, "I have this opportunity to host the Girls' Teen Summit at a larger facility. I'm going to need a lot of help putting on this event because I have never had it on a Saturday."

Sandy looked at me and said, "Absolutely not!"

---

[2] Aleks Kajstura, "States of Women's Incarceration: The Global Context 2018," *Prison Policy Initiative* (June 2018): https://www.prisonpolicy.org/global/women/2018.html.

I was shocked and thought to myself, "Umm…maybe she didn't hear me." I asked her again.

She stopped what she was doing and gave me a very stern look. Rudely, she said, "I told you, I'm not helping you plan the Summit. I said it before and I mean it, so don't ask me again!"

At that moment, I felt frozen in time. Every hurtful childhood memory of rejection and feeling unloved began to surface. I wanted to bite back at her and say, "How dare you say no and come at me like that after everything I have done for you! I've provided speakers for your conference! I donated my time and door prizes so you could have successful events, and you sit there and snap at me?"

I was steaming and beyond angry, to say the least. I felt used and thrown away like trash. Sandy had gotten all she could get out of me. I was going to give her a piece of my mind. Then the Holy Spirit stopped me. He said, "Be quiet and don't say a word. You tell her you understand and walk out."

I thought, "What?" The Holy Spirit instructed me again, and I did as I was told. When I left, she didn't look at me; she just kept doing her work.

I walked out of the room perplexed, crushed, and hurt. The Holy Spirit then said, "Next year, you're going to help her with her conference as you have done every year. I want you to go beyond what you have done in the past. You will be humble, help her with excellence, and put your A-game on!!"

Back at my car, I sat stunned, but trusted the Holy Spirit's guidance. I knew I had been given wisdom to handle this situation.

Her response brought up the past pain, rejection, and disappointments I had endured throughout my childhood. When anger rises up in us, it is often a secondary response to our primary emotions. My childhood had instilled a primary feeling of rejection.

The next year, I followed the Holy Spirit's advice. I helped her with a smile and didn't expect her to change her mind about my Summit.

Fast forward to the summer of 2017. Out of the blue, Sandy called me. It was early in the morning, and the first thing she said was, "Congratulations! You're 2018 Woman of the Year!"

I said, "Huh? What did you say?"

She said it again. "You're 2018 Woman of the Year, and I want to extend my congratulations to you."

I said, "There is no mention of this on social media, and I haven't seen any news release. How do you know I'm Woman of the Year?"

"I know because I sit on the committee. You had several nominations. They asked me, 'Is Premadonna really doing all this work in the community?' I told them, 'Yes—not only does she host her Girls' Teen Summit, she also helps me with my conference for the youth. She does an excellent job!'"

My jaw dropped. I was completely taken back at receiving such a distinguished award.

The lesson I learned from this is, I should not allow my past pain to affect my future. I could have given into past hurts and said words to Sandy I would have regretted. Instead, I heeded the wisdom of the Holy Spirit. Because of my obedience, I was one of ten women awarded Pinnacle Woman of the year by Tulsa YWCA and the Mayor's Commission on the Status of Women.

Many times, we remain stuck in past offenses. This can cause us to have poor relationships with friends, significant others, and co-workers. I encourage you to allow Proverbs 4:5-8 to guide you throughout your life. As verse 6 says, "Do not forsake wisdom, and she will protect you; love her, and she will watch over you."

Pray.

Lord, You know more than I possibly could. You know what's going on with the people I meet, and You know my heart pretty well, too. Help me to hear Your voice over my own emotions. I promise to listen and obey.

Think.

We can't change our past hurts, but the enemy delights when we live in response to them. He wants us to stay stuck and spiritually unhealthy. Focus on the present. What can you do to make healthy decisions about your relationships with friends, family, a significant other, or co-workers?

Act.

Think of a painful memory that has stifled you from being all God has called you to be. I'd like you to take that painful memory and give it to Jesus right now. Ask Him to pour His blood across that memory and give you the mind of Christ.

Day 12: Difficult People

by Kristi Bridges

Galatians 6 NLT

[4] Pay careful attention to your own work, for then you will get the satisfaction of a job well done, and you won't need to compare yourself to anyone else. [5] For we are each responsible for our own conduct.

Psalm 118 NLT

[6] The LORD is for me, so I will have no fear. What can mere people do to me?

[7] Yes, the LORD is for me; he will help me. I will look in triumph at those who hate me.

Proverbs 22 NLT

[24] Don't befriend angry people or associate with hot-tempered people,

[25] or you will learn to be like them and endanger your soul.

"You're so sweet," he said. I'm sure he meant it as a compliment, but what my heart heard was the unspoken, "I don't love you." In hindsight, it was a good thing. We had very different destinies, but when I was with him, I lost sight of my dreams and acted in ways I later regretted.

Some people make us forget who we are. They may light up our hearts until like moths, we hover near their flames and toast our wings. In a misdirected romance, it's best to cut ties. When dating or flirting with someone who is clearly on a different path, it helps to think of them as someone else's future spouse. Say goodbye instead of creating baggage for both of you. Jesus came to give you abundant life. Trust Him.

Other people simply push our buttons until we lose ourselves to juvenile attitudes or old patterns. It's hardest with relatives and people we grew up around, but God uses these challenging relationships to develop us. If we cut ties, we may end up in a similar relationship because there's something we're supposed to be learning, a skill we're meant to acquire. Maybe the skill is how to choose better companions, but most of the time it has to do with being our true, God-built selves in every situation.

Who are you on the inside, the person you believe yourself to be? What do you show online and in new relationships? Is that inner person honest, kind, generous, wise? Of course! How can you be that person in every situation?

Charge up.   Charge your battery by spending the majority of your time with God and people who bring out your best self. That sounds easy, but it's important. Jesus had one disciple who ended up betraying Him, but He had eleven who were faithful friends. He also communed alone with the Father on a regular basis.

Tune up.   Sprinkle in short times with the person who challenges you. You must practice dealing with them. The prettiest guitar looks perfect while it's being admired in the case. Only by plucking do we discover the out-of-tune strings. That difficult person is simply finding your flat strings. Once you're tuned up and good at dealing with them, the Holy Spirit can make beautiful music of your life.

Listen up. When you're together, give this person your attention. Sometimes people are annoying, fearful, crotchety, or make bad decisions just because they need attention. Stay off your phone, don't sit and watch TV. Instead, ask a question about something which interests them. I've found getting people to tell stories about their lives or projects, favorite movies or books can change the dynamic of our interactions. If you encounter resistance, say, "I feel like we're a little disconnected, and I want to change that."

Colossians 4:6 NIV says, "Let your conversation be always full of grace, seasoned with salt, so that you may know how to answer everyone." God gives us grace every day. That means we should be giving grace as well. How did Jesus treat the flirtatious woman at the well or the rich man who asked how to get to heaven but didn't want to help the poor? We might have been tempted to flirt back or nag them. We might have talked to them in a dismissive or sarcastic manner, but Jesus knew those techniques don't work. Instead, He maintained an awareness of who He was and was kind without being fake. That takes practice!

Reiterate. Salt makes things taste good, and it's a preservative. When you hit the flavor that gets your person talking, reiterate some of what they've said. This shows you're listening and makes them feel cared for.

Talk straight. Be graceful but direct when expressing your needs. For example, if someone is constantly reminding you of who you once were, manipulating you, or talking negatively about other people, you might say, "I'd rather talk about something else." It will take practice to avoid blowing up or shutting down. Try it with someone safe, a supportive friend who will give you good feedback.

Name the place.   Avoid habits which prevent you from being taken seriously. Sarcasm and zingers—joking insults—seem funny but sound passive-aggressive. Also, avoid being indecisive. When someone asks where you'd like to eat, even if you don't care, just name a place. Passivity can turn a friendly moment into a struggle. Simplicity is power.

Bring a date.   Remember you're not God. Is there someone in your life who is abusive or dangerous? Is there someone with whom you always end up doing things you wish you hadn't? We want to be godly, and we're becoming stronger every day, but we aren't God. If someone is destructive and not just difficult, break off the relationship. If you must be around them, bring someone who is strong in faith and will have your back. When Jesus sent the disciples out to heal and deliver people from demons, He sent them in pairs.

Pray.

Lord, thank You for loving me and this difficult person. I am so grateful You don't expect me to be perfect, yet! I like the changes You're making in me, and I want to keep them even when I'm around this person. I'm sorry for times I've failed. Please forgive me and grab my tongue whenever I'm tempted to fall into old patterns. I expect to see change only You can bring. In Jesus's Name, amen.

Think.

How many faith-building, wise people do you have in your circle? Which of them would offer good feedback and prayer support for dealing with this difficult person?

Act.

Write down three things your difficult person finds interesting. Write something simple you might say if the conversation becomes dangerous. Rehearse each of these and pray before visiting this person.

Day 13: Recruited for the JFL

by Smiley Elmore, Jr. PhD

John 3:30 NIV

He must become greater; I must become less.

In the closet of the two-bedroom apartment I shared with my new wife, I held a knife to my throat. In the back of my mind, I heard Momma's voice, "Son, God made you special! He has something bigger for you than pro football! DON'T GIVE UP!"

In high school, I was an All-State running back, recruited by several big colleges in the US. I chose Wichita State University, where I was on a football scholarship. Just before the end of my first semester, WSU dropped its football program. I was recruited again, this time by even bigger colleges. I accepted another scholarship at the University of Missouri (Mizzou).

I worked extremely hard, and in my debut game as a junior, I had one of the greatest games of my life. I gained 187 yards on eighteen carries. This placed me fifth on the "Best Performances in the School's History" list. ESPN talked about me. Fans wrote, wishing me luck in winning the prestigious Heisman Trophy, awarded at season's end to the best college football player in the country. I was second leading player in the nation behind the great Barry Sanders. Barry was the running back who would later win that award.

I read my newspaper articles and listened to what fans were saying about how great I was. NFL was in my future. I became conceited and began relying on myself and not Jesus Christ, to whom I'd committed my life when I was an adolescent. I placed my beautiful, all-satisfying relationship with Christ in the backseat of my '77 Cutlass Supreme and chose the disgusting, finite peanuts of the world as His replacement.

After defeating our cross-state rival, Kansas State University, my teammates and I celebrated with a steak dinner. In the middle of my meal, I noticed I didn't have enough butter to finish my bread. I politely called our waiter over, "Sir, I don't have enough butter to finish my meal. Can you please bring me another pat of butter?"

The waiter smiled. "Young man, it's restaurant policy to provide only two pats of butter per person. So sorry, I can't bring you any more butter."

I laughed, "Sir, do you know who I am?! My name is Smiley Elmore, Jr. I'm Mizzou Tigers football star! I'm in the school's record books. You'll be watching me on TV on Sundays when I make it to the NFL. Did you know that?"

The waiter smiled again. "No sir, I didn't know that. But, do you know who I am, young man?"

"No, how could I know who you are?" I replied.

The waiter said, "I'm the guy in charge of the butter, and you ain't getting anymore!"

It was downhill from there as I steadily took my eyes off of Jesus. I even began to question my existence as a Christian. I turned my back on God and started doing things my dad and mom would never approve of, let alone my Savior, Jesus Christ.

Raised in church, I gave my life to Christ at twelve years old. So, I knew I was wrong. But I thought since I was behaving better than many of my teammates, I was okay. I thought since I only said two or three cuss words a day, compared to my teammates' countless cuss words, I was all good. I only drank wine coolers on Wednesday nights. My friends drank hard liquor Wednesday and Saturday nights, so I was great. I only had two girlfriends, on opposite sides of campus. My teammates had two and three girlfriends in the same dorm building (and sometimes the same dorm room). That meant I was good, right?

I tore my knee ligament, and my NFL football dreams drifted away. Depression set in, as I graduated from college with no NFL teams contacting me. I went on to graduate school and played two summers in the professional Arena Football League. After many doors were slammed in my face by NFL scouts, I was ready to spill what remained of my life on the closet floor. My hand paused.

"DON'T GIVE UP! Come back to God! Come back to God! COME BACK TO GOD!" My mom's words rang louder and louder. The words from letters she'd sent me for a year finally sank into her oldest son's mind and heart. I threw that knife down, and I became a REAL man. A real man is not the one with twenty-one-inch biceps who cusses his wife out, puts his fist through a wall, and gets kicked out. No, a real man is the one who gets on his knees and commits his life to Jesus Christ! That's a real man.

In that closet, the Lord completely turned my life around. He miraculously restored my marriage. Since that day, God's taken me around the globe, speaking life to millions of young people and performing feats of strength in school assemblies and churches. Maybe I didn't make it to the NFL–the National Football League but I made it to the greatest league of all. I'm in the JFL, the JESUS FOREVER LEAGUE!

Pray.

Jesus, You demonstrated confidence everywhere You went. You were never proud, telling Your disciples in John 5:19 NLT, "I tell you the truth, the Son can do nothing by himself. He does only what he sees the Father doing. Whatever the Father does, the Son also does." Confidence without pride is something I'd like to learn. Holy Spirit, please hold me back when I start to be proud and lift me up when I need to be confident. Above all, remind me every day God always has a plan, no matter what surprises life brings. In Jesus's Name, amen.

Think.

It's wise to picture your goals. Maybe you'd like to win a Heisman trophy. Imagine your goal right now. Then imagine it as a tourist attraction on the side of a highway. You are eternal, with a life which will carry you far beyond that one goal. Work hard for it but keep your faith in our eternal Creator.

Act.

Have you ever gotten a "big head"—a feeling that everyone should recognize your importance? Perhaps you've been a star of some sort, or maybe you were simply working on a class project and had a strong idea of how things should be done. If you acted pridefully, it might be worthwhile to apologize for your behavior. You don't have to be self-deprecating. The ability to apologize honestly and humbly is an extremely attractive quality.

Day 14: God Doesn't Lie

by Dr. Philip Greenaway

Numbers 23:19 NLT

God is not human, that he should lie, not a human being, that he should change his mind. Does he speak and then not act? Does he promise and not fulfill?

One badge of fishermen is stretching the truth. "That fish was a monster!" they'll say. It is an anomaly that the greatest fisherman who ever lived, Jesus Christ, who said, "Follow me, and I will make you fishers of men," never told a lie (Matthew 4:19 NKV). Jesus was God and there is one little thing about God that is unquestionably true: He cannot lie. He can no more lie than a chicken can open a Facebook account!

His perfect truthfulness is perhaps one of the most wonderful things about God. It is also the reason His Word is utterly unbreakable. As the Creator who spoke the worlds into being, He can't go back on His word. If He did, the course of all things natural and divine would be altered. If He were ever found to have stretched the truth in even the smallest detail, everything He has ever said would be suspect. But we needn't worry because that is not only improbable, it is also impossible!

My father once told me about his kid brother Melvin, who grew up playing the trumpet in the church orchestra. Melvin was called into the ministry as a young man, but then World War II came. Like other boys in other generations, he found himself thrust into the midst of a conflict. The horrors of that war were so complete that after the war, Melvin never darkened the door of a church again. He married and had four sons.

My father and his family wept for Melvin's soul. The one person they thought would be devastated by Melvin's refusal to follow God was his mother. Surprisingly, she never faltered in her calm assurance that somehow, some way, Melvin would be saved.

My father would call his mom and invariably Melvin's salvation would come up. Dad would ask, "Mom, what do you think?"

She would answer, "My boy's going to make it."

"But how do you know, Mom?"

Then would come the standard reply–not the automatic response of robot faith, but the declaration of a fact that was as real to her as if it had already come to pass. "Son, God doesn't lie, and you never quit believing!"

Five, ten, seventeen years went by. My father was walking out of his office headed for Europe on a mission trip, when he heard the frantic footsteps of his secretary running after him. She stopped him. "There's a call you need to take."

The voice on the other end of the line told him, "Your brother Melvin dropped dead this morning." My father hung his head and cried. His tears weren't for himself or for Melvin– it was too late for that. His tears were for a mother who had believed her son was going to turn back to God before it was too late.

Instead of flying to Europe, Dad flew to Boston. He drove to the mortuary. He leaned over to kiss his brother's cold brow and began to weep uncontrollably. Feeling someone by his side, he looked around and came face to face with Melvin's wife. She said, "Come over here. I want to tell you something. I don't know much about these things, but last night your brother said goodnight to the boys and went to his room. He didn't get into bed. He did something I didn't know Melvin could do. He fell on his knees and began to pray. Then he lifted his hands. Then he wept. A few hours later, he got into his car to head for work, turned the key, and slumped over the steering wheel, dead."

Dad ran to the telephone. He called his mom and said, "Melvin's dead, Mom, but it's not all bad!"

"I know it," she said.

"What do you know, Mom?"

She said, "My boy made it."

Dad said, "How do you know?"

"Son," she said, "how many times do I have to tell you: God doesn't lie, and you never quit believing!"

Do you feel forsaken by God? At the beginning of a trial, you had friends to bear the load, and the Lord seemed to confirm things to you daily. Now it's been some time since you felt His presence. Doubt is seeping in, and fears are piling up. Maybe bitterness is hanging around. You no longer understand why you're having to take this pressure for so long without relief.

Perhaps that is how the psalmist felt as he penned the words of Psalm 42:1-3, 9-10 NLT:

¹As the deer longs for streams of water, so I long for you, O God. ²I thirst for God, the living God. When can I go and stand before him? ³Day and night, I have only tears for food, while my enemies continually taunt me, saying, "Where is this God of yours?"

⁹"O God my rock," I cry, "Why have you forgotten me? Why must I wander around in grief, oppressed by my enemies?"

¹⁰Their taunts break my bones. They scoff, "Where is this God of yours?"

The details aren't spelled out, but the author of those words is in deep distress. Yet, this is one who has experience with God. He finishes Psalm 42 with a statement of faith in such contrast to his surrounding gloom, it lightens the landscape like a sharp lighthouse beam cutting through the foggy night of the soul.

[11]Why am I discouraged? Why is my heart so sad? I will put my hope in God! I will praise him again – my Savior and my God!

Pray.

Father, I come to You believing that you cannot lie. Please strengthen my faith so that I never quit believing.

Think.

When you started kindergarten, you knew one day, you'd graduate. Did it happen the next day? The next year? Were there times you wanted to quit school and never go back? Write down five differences between the person you are now and the person you were on your first day of school.

Act.

This week, when you encounter a challenge, ask God how He'd like to use this situation to develop you or your future. If you're praying for someone, give God your tongue. Say only what God is saying, no more and no less.

Week 3: Hold on Tight!

Day 15: Tough Stuff

by Kristi Bridges

Psalm 18 NLT

[19] He led me to a place of safety; he rescued me because he delights in me... [25] To the faithful you show yourself faithful; to those with integrity you show integrity. [26] To the pure you show yourself pure, but to the crooked you show yourself shrewd. [27] You rescue the humble, but you humiliate the proud. [28] You light a lamp for me. The Lord, my God, lights up my darkness... [32] God arms me with strength, and he makes my way perfect. [33] He makes me as surefooted as a deer, enabling me to stand on mountain heights. [34] He trains my hands for battle; he strengthens my arm to draw a bronze bow.

God likes you. The first verse of today's selection might sound a little arrogant: "He rescued me because He delights in me." Seriously? Yep. When God made Adam, He wanted a companion to walk in the garden with Him. That's never changed. He made you because He specifically wanted a Y.O.U. He delights in you and enjoys showing off for you.

One fall, I was in Des Moines teaching a class. I never expected Iowa to be so pretty, but there I was on the way to my hotel, and I couldn't stop ooh-ing and aah-ing. The trees were straight out of a Bob Ross painting. They were sunshine yellow, crayon red, and deep purple, and they nuzzled cat-like against heavy, blue-grey clouds. I said, "Lord, You do great work!"

Who doesn't like to hear that?

David says, "To the faithful, you show yourself faithful…to the pure you show yourself pure." I would add: To the appreciative, our Creator shows so much more. Psalm 37:4 NLT tells us, "Take delight in the Lord, and he will give you your heart's desires." Your Maker knows your heart better than you do. He enjoys fulfilling desires you didn't even realize you had.

One of the craziest myths about God is that He'll keep us from going through hard times. Some people think if they're perfect enough, they can reinforce His protection and be completely wrapped in airtight bubbles of safety. When those people get hurt, they decide God is a myth. That's not the way relationships work, even a relationship with God.

Let's say you and I were friends, and I decided you should do my math homework. Maybe that didn't line up with your values, but you picked me up when my car broke down and shared your free movie passes with me. If I failed math, would it be logical for me to decide you didn't exist? Instead of turning away from you, it would make more sense for me to enjoy your friendship. I might even mature a little in the process.

In today's Psalm, David told the story of running for his life from a homicidal king. David is described as a man after God's own heart because he pursued a relationship with God in every season of his life. What did he get? Light for the way, strength for the battle, stamina for the long trek. Jesus himself said in John 16:33b NLT, "Here on earth you will have many trials and sorrows. But take heart, because I have overcome the world."

You and I are not living in heaven yet. We are living in a world that desperately needs Jesus, because when they're not following Him, people do awful things to each other. The writers of this devotional have experienced some rough stuff, but we live in triumph because we each have a personal relationship with the One who made us, the same God who walked with David and sent us Jesus.

I recently had a deep conversation with a former soldier who had been much too close to the horrors people do. He's one of the wisest, most compassionate people I know, but he's missing out on an incredible relationship with his Maker, because he believes that if God were real and He were good, He'd never have created anyone who might possibly do evil.

I've only been alive a few decades, so I'm not going to try to explain God's motivations, but I know a few things. I can tell He exists. He's been around longer than me, and if He never created anyone who might hurt someone else, He wouldn't have made me. I'm happy to be alive to tell you how awesome He is. God is good, and He can turn dirt clods into diamonds when we turn to Him.

What about you? Have you ever doubted God because of the evil you've seen? You've grown up watching fellow students get shot and parents break each other's hearts. Maybe you've been through personal horrors you're not ready to talk about. Many of us have. Let God be the source of everything you need. Whether He gives you protection or stamina, He'll never leave your side. The results will be incredible.

Are you still wondering? Perhaps someone gave you this book, but the Jesus story doesn't make sense to you. Would you be willing to suspend your disbelief, this month?

Pray.

God, I don't know what to believe. They say You let us murder Your son in order to save us from our sins. This world is pretty messed up if we can torture and kill a man who did nothing but help people, so I can see how we might need saving. But none of it lines up with my experience of the world. I confess I have a couple of decades of experience with a few hundred people in a single realm of existence. If it's true that Jesus was crucified and rose from the dead, so I could have a relationship with You, would You please connect with me this month? I'd like to know You personally.

In Jesus's name, amen.

Think.

When have you discovered strength you didn't know you had or experienced clarity when you didn't know which way to go?

Act.

This week, ask people what life challenges they've overcome. Notice the difference between those who hold onto bitterness and those who live in gratitude.

Day 16: Midnight Meditation

by Cyndilu Miller

Psalm 63:6-8 ESV

*[6]When I remember You on my bed, and
meditate on You in the night watches,*

*[7]For You have been my help, and in the shadow
of Your wings I sing for joy.*

[8]My soul clings to You; Your right hand upholds me.

I lay awake, eyes staring into the darkness. Would I always
be alone? Had I messed up my life forever? My thoughts
swirled, sleep seemed far away. One baby cried in the next
room, one baby kicked from within. Have I really done this
again? I thought.

"First time's a mistake, second time's your own fault," my
dad had said. Was he right? He didn't know all that I had
experienced. How could he know? I had so much pushed down
inside, hidden from everyone, including my own self. This was
the only way I could get through. Abuse took away my self-
worth. The baby in the next room and the one within were my
reasons to keep living. Because of them, I kept reaching for the
love of God.

I meditate on You in the night watches…

Meditation was not something I grew up understanding.
When I was eighteen, I met the one who would become my
lifelong best friend. That first night I stayed at her house, she
walked me through her evening prayer routine. It is so simple.

Close your eyes and say, "I love you God," in quietness. "I allow You to lift me up into Your eternal presence." Then we simply lay in silence, focusing on those thoughts.

Godly meditation is the gift I want to give you today. By the end of this short devotional, I want you to know that God loves you. He is waiting for you to quiet yourself and climb under the shadow of His wings. From there, you may sing for joy as you cling to God. He will hold you up!

In the night seasons of my life, I was so far from God that I could not see Him at work. Even then, when I would lie down to sleep, my spirit and my soul cried out. There was a knowing in my spirit that God was somehow watching out for me, a knowing that God was there even in the middle of the turmoil that had become my life.

Being a teen mother was not my dream, but it was my reality. With a first baby by seventeen and a second at nineteen, I found myself living a life I had not planned. I was caught in an abusive relationship which would lead me down an even more painful road. At times, I wished death would swallow me up and other times, I wanted to walk away from everything.

I loved my children so very much. I thought I was ready to be a mother. In reality, I was just making the best of it. Looking at the bright side helped to keep me sane during the times abuse or dismay would threaten to overtake me. In those midnight meditations, I found a way out through the power of God and His word for my life. I took refuge in the hope that nothing can separate us from the love of God!

Romans 8:35-39 NLT

[35]Can anything ever separate us from Christ's love? Does it mean he no longer loves us if we have trouble or calamity, or are persecuted, or hungry, or destitute, or in danger, or

threatened with death? ³⁶(As the Scriptures say, "For your sake we are killed every day; we are being slaughtered like sheep.") ³⁷No, despite all these things, overwhelming victory is ours through Christ, who loved us. ³⁸And I am convinced that nothing can ever separate us from God's love. Neither death nor life, neither angels nor demons, neither our fears for today nor our worries about tomorrow—not even the powers of hell can separate us from God's love. ³⁹No power in the sky above or in the earth below—indeed, nothing in all creation will ever be able to separate us from the love of God that is revealed in Christ Jesus our Lord.

Pray.

Dear God, even when I don't feel it, You are with me. We are here together even when my soul is dark. Thank You for being a light for me in the darkness. You take me as I am, showing me I'm loved no matter what! Be with me in this minute and carry me to the next one too. In Jesus's name, amen.

Think.

God gave people the freedom of choice and that means they hurt us sometimes. He gives us the choice to seek comfort in Him and trust Him to lead us through. Can you remember a time when things seemed dark? Are you more capable, loving, or wise now? If you're still going through a dark time, or if you're still carrying scars, ask God to be your shelter and healer. Make sure to spend time with Him, allowing Him to do what you're asking.

Act.

If you wake in the night this week, or if you find yourself feeling dark on the inside, try this. It's a simple meditative exercise, called a Breath Prayer.

1. Sit up straight but relaxed. You'll sleep better if you stay awake for this.
2. Breathe in slowly.
3. As you breathe out, say, "Hi, Lord."
4. Breathe in slowly.
5. As you breathe out, say, "I love you."
6. Breathe in slowly.
7. Breathe out a line from one of today's Scriptures, such as, "Nothing separates me from Your love."
8. Repeat the process a few more times, using the same line.
9. Ask God if there's anything He'd like to say to you.
10. You should be able to sleep peacefully. If you are still awake, just talk to God. He never sleeps.

Day 17: The One Who Heals Me

by Pastor Jimmy John Sills

Mark 1 NLT

[40] A man with leprosy came and knelt in front of Jesus, begging to be healed. "If you are willing, you can heal me and make me clean," he said. [41] Moved with compassion, Jesus reached out and touched him. "I am willing," he said. "Be healed!"

I am amazed at the lengths that our adversary will go to deplete our drive and ambition, darken our attitude, distance us from God, and diminish the reflection of His character in us – all to destroy our soul. God doesn't want that.

I was born to an unwed mother. The inconvenience of my existence was handled by passing me off to an adoption agency where I was placed with a loving family. They were eager and anxious to have a little boy, but they were also too scared to know what they were doing.

When I was nine, a trusted individual molested me. Our family decided to bury the secret. My hurt and feelings of shame and guilt were never addressed and always avoided. This burial technique became a pattern in my life. After all, my birth mother "buried" her shame by sending me away. My adoptive parents "buried" my molestation by never addressing it in public or with medical professionals.

I had heard the gospel of Jesus. I wanted to know this man who would accept me as I was, take away my hurt, and heal my broken heart. I could not fathom that anyone could exist who could do these things. "I am willing; be healed," Jesus said. It was more than I could imagine.

Hope is often hard to imagine. We want to believe but dismiss it as unattainable. We decide we are unworthy to be considered eligible for God's love. Our histories or thoughts are too dark.

Satan is a liar.

Think about someone who has never experienced the sun. It's incomprehensible. "Our planet journeys in orbit around it," you might say. "It rises in the east and sets in the west. It stays longer on summer days and warms the air. It paints the sky with pink and orange and purple as it sets." Someone who had never seen it would have a hard time imagining an object which rises, sets, warms, and paints.

God's love, acceptance, and assurance are incomprehensible to someone who has never known Him. In Plato's Republic is a story called the "Allegory of the Cave." Plato begins the story by having the audience imagine a cave where people are imprisoned from birth.

These prisoners are chained, so that they can only see a dark cave wall. The way out is behind them, as well as the bonfire and sun. Condemned to see only what is before them, they hear their captors conduct day-to-day activities, and they see shadows on the wall, but that is it. Satan wants us to hear only what he and our captors say and to see in a diminished or distorted way.

In Plato's allegory, one of the prisoners escapes and makes it outside to a vibrant world of color and life. The prisoner is overwhelmed, squinting, frightened. Free from captors and chains, he returns to the mouth of the cave for a moment. It's the only security he's known. Soon, the desire to explore takes over.

New life lies ahead…

Imagine this beauty, novelty, boldness of life in comparison to the dank and shadowy half-life of the cave. How many times do we become free, delivered from darkness and doubt, only to be drawn back little by little to the way of life we know?

As the days pass, our ex-prisoner returns to tell others of this wonderful new world. The prisoners are shocked. They hear of freedom, the ability to move unencumbered and experience the sun. Flowers, trees, fish in streams—it's too much to comprehend. *The ex-prisoner must have lost his mind,* they think. *Perhaps he's a phantasm sent to confuse and torture us.* They will never leave the security of the shadowy world they know.

Our adversary wants us to accept a "less than" life—an unconfronted captor, a buried consequence. He knows time does not heal all wounds. He knows just as a pot of water on a fire will come to a boil, rage will erupt like a poison, scalding everything around it. When the water is gone and the fire is burned down, the pot is scorched, dry and warped.

As long as we face the wall, hurts and hopes buried, we see a perverted world, broken and tormented. We hear but see nothing clearly except what plays on the wall. Isn't it time to walk out of the cave? Ask Jesus to free you and heal your broken heart. Ask Him to help you forgive and live a life of grace and mercy.

Psalm 147:3 NLT

He heals the broken hearted and bandages their wounds.

I was a prisoner. Buried circumstances shaped my life. Unchallenged hurts, unforgiven captors, unwitting participants made shadows of hurt, rage, and shame on the wall of my "less than" life. I hungered for new life, but rejected it, unable to break free. I would rather stay in the comfort of my familiar broken condition than escape to this incomprehensible "more than" life.

- Yes, it is uncomfortable when you first come out of the darkness.
- Yes, it is difficult to navigate the world of new opportunities.
- Yes, it can hurt, as you long for the familiarity of the life you once knew.

But there was hope – wonderful hope. God is the one who sees us even when we cannot see for ourselves. He will lead you from that dark cave, if you only ask. He is willing.

Psalm 30:2 NIV

Lord my God, I called to you for help, and you have healed me.

A final encouragement. Once you know about this world of abundant life, you might experience a call back to the cave when storms come. Don't go back. Call on Jesus, your faithful friend. He is closer than a brother, a whisper away.

He was there for the disciples in Mark 4. As their tiny fishing boat in the lake of Galilee was being violently tossed on the waves of an incoming storm, they cried out. Jesus calmed the storm. As the disciples shook and trembled, He asked, "Why did you worry? Was I not here?" Call on Him today.

Pray.

Jesus, examine my heart. Expose what has been buried in me to Your light. Take away the hate, rage, shame, guilt, uncertainty, and blame. Reveal the me I was created to be. You said You are willing to heal. I am willing to let You. I'll hold tight to Your promises and let go of the cave mind, even when freedom seems unattainable.

Think.

List the things that diminish your walk with God – the shadows that keep you in a "less than" life. Then read this Scripture and imagine those things are causing the waves on this troubled sea. Jesus is with you, resting and inviting you to do the same. No matter what is going on around you, replace angry, anxious, bitter thoughts with gratitude that He is here. Trust and rest.

Mark 4 NIV

[35] *That day when evening came, he said to his disciples, "Let us go over to the other side."* [36] *Leaving the crowd behind, they took him along, just as he was, in the boat. There were also other boats with him.* [37] *A furious squall came up, and the waves broke over the boat, so that it was nearly swamped.* [38] *Jesus was in the stern, sleeping on a cushion. The disciples woke him and said to him, "Teacher, don't you care if we drown?"*

[39] *He got up, rebuked the wind and said to the waves, "Quiet! Be still!" Then the wind died down and it was completely calm.* [40] *He said to his disciples, "Why are you so afraid? Do you still have no faith?"*

Act.

What's more important?

a. Your desire to appear perfect as long as you can hold it together.

b. God's desire to make you whole for life.

Give God space to do the work of healing you. It may take time away from other things, but the lasting impact will be worthwhile. Find at least two godly people to pray you through the storm. This will give you a balance of counsel and avoid strain on your friendships. If you need a professional counselor, get one. God has called people to that position for times like this.

Day 18: Egg Escape

by Kim White

Philippians 4 NLT

[19] And this same God who takes care of me will supply all your needs from his glorious riches, which have been given to us in Christ Jesus.

"Ma'am, would you step outside?"

I looked at the officer, not quite understanding and not sure what to do. Why was he here? The question didn't sound like a choice, so I followed him out.

"Shut the door, please," he said. I obeyed. "What's going on?" he asked.

"Nothing!" I replied. "I didn't call the police. Are you sure you're at the right house?"

He looked at me knowingly and said, "Your son called. He told the 911 operator, 'I think my daddy is killing my mommy.' Know anything about that?"

I was mortified. Every night, I put my boys to bed before their father got home. I tried to remain quiet as I battled his rage alone. I didn't know my son could even hear us.

"You don't have to do *that* anymore," the officer said.

"What?" I asked, as though I could keep him from knowing what he clearly understood.

He handed me his card. "Call me when you're ready."

You don't have to do that anymore. The words were etched on the insides of my eyelids as I tried to sleep. In the morning, they floated on the bathroom mirror. *You don't have to do that anymore.* But what would I do?

When I was five years old, I played a game with my cousins. I was the store owner, and they had to buy whatever I sold. It was pretend, but I knew one day I'd be the boss of my own business. I was an entrepreneur from the time I was born. At sixteen, I owned a furniture store. It wasn't as much fun as I'd anticipated. My friends went out and had fun, but I had to work. Owning a furniture store wasn't for me, but I still dreamed of a big office with lots of employees and nobody telling me what to do.

I pulled the officer's card from its hiding place. I had changed. Nights of fighting for my life and dignity made me forget who I was and the talents God had given me. *You don't have to do that anymore.* What else could I do? I didn't even have a vehicle, and we lived out in the country. "Lord, what are You expecting me to do?"

God said, "What do you have?" I looked around. I had chickens. Chickens had eggs, so pretty soon I had a business. When eggs were at the store for $.69 a dozen, my eggs brought $3.00. My chickens were hand-raised and healthy, the best in the entire world! People were happy to pay, and one day I had enough egg money to buy a truck.

I strapped my son into the seatbelt, just before my husband drove up. He came at me and managed to get my door open. From the look on his face, I knew if he got me out of the truck, my boys and I would die that day. I shifted to reverse and sped down the driveway. I didn't care if he kept the door, we were going. He lost his grip, so I spun the truck around and floored it. That night, I lay my boys down to sleep on a cardboard box I'd flattened to protect them from the cold concrete floor. We lived in an old warehouse until I earned enough to rent an apartment.

God gives us the resources we need. Even when we stop dreaming, He doesn't. Selling those eggs reminded me of who I was. Eventually, I had my own oil business, complete with the big office full of employees I dreamed of as a little girl. There are some intimidating men in the oil business, but they were nothing compared to the one I escaped. Today, I coach entrepreneurs and executives with the lessons I've learned.

Think back to when you were young. Did you see clues to your gifts? Are you currently doing things which light you up and make you feel good about yourself? Are you curious and ready to make things happen?

Or are you trying to keep a good face in areas where you feel weak? Are you fighting your way alone, through a circumstance or relationship that's stealing your life? You aren't truly alone. God has given you the resources you need. You might have to eliminate the word "Can't" from your vocabulary in order to see how those resources can be used. When you are ready for a change, God will bridge the distance with people who can help.

Remember my furniture store? Have you ever thought you wanted something, but when you got it, it wasn't that great? That's happened to me with a few businesses I've owned. Bring value to others while you examine what you'd like to continue and what you'd like to stop. You might have to finish learning a skill or fulfill your commitments before moving on. Don't worry—we grow with every experience, if we're willing.

Pray.

Lord, thank You for holding my future in Your hands. If I'm overlooking my resources or talents, I'm sorry. Please point them out to me, and I'll work diligently to get out of any place I feel stuck.

Think.

You don't have to do that anymore. Are you feeling trapped in any way?

Act.

Talk to God first and then talk to a wise friend about what you can do to move forward. Proverbs 15:22 NLT says, "Plans go wrong for lack of advice; many advisers bring success."

Day 19: Boundaries

by Kristi Bridges

2 Corinthians 9 NLT

[7] You must each decide in your heart how much to give. And don't give reluctantly or in response to pressure. "For God loves a person who gives cheerfully." [8] And God will generously provide all you need. Then you will always have everything you need and plenty left over to share with others.

Ephesians 4:16 NLT

He makes the whole body fit together perfectly. As each part does its own special work, it helps the other parts grow, so that the whole body is healthy and growing and full of love.

I'll never forget the time I asked my grandparents for a loan and they said no. I was shocked. Sure, I'd borrowed $2000 and hadn't made the promised payments, but times were tough. Something was always going wrong and adulting is expensive. Paying back the $2000 took a few years. I made sporadic payments whenever I felt I could—occasionally using the Christmas and birthday money they freely gave.

Without them to rescue me, I learned to budget so I could handle things that came up. Once I paid off the grands, I even began to save a little bit, although it took a while to keep my savings. There was always some emergency or other, until I made tithing and saving automatic.

I'll also never forget the time I stopped speaking to one of my longest-term friends for six months. Bipolar, she'd taught me much about the human psyche and compassion, but one day I realized that those closest to her, including myself, had crippled her with compassion. We had tried to help her but rendered her helpless. I couldn't bring myself to answer any more hour-long, emotionally exhausting phone calls. I hated myself for abandoning her and was miserable that I couldn't fix her pain. In desperation I wondered if I'd done her wrong when I stopped her from committing suicide a few years before.

I believe it is always right to stop someone from suicide when possible, and I'm happy my friend is alive today. The problem was not that she had lived. The problem was that neither my friend nor I understood personal responsibility and boundaries.

I had looked at the sacrifice Jesus made on the cross and thought I understood selfless, unconditional love. During counseling, I came to a life-altering epiphany. Jesus gave Himself when we didn't deserve it, but our response is required. He did His part and offered us the opportunity to do ours.

His whole ministry demonstrated this balance. When He met Zaccheus, His friendly, righteous presence inspired Zaccheus to live an honest life. The ten lepers had to start walking before they received the healing Jesus promised. Luke 17:14 NIV says, "When he saw them, he said to them, 'Go and show yourselves to the priests.' And as they went, they were cleansed." When He called His disciples, He said, "Follow me."

It is impossible for us to enjoy truly abundant life without stepping up to the challenge of living. If I'd remained dependent on my grandparents, our relationship would have been based on them bailing me out. They might have become resentful, and I would have missed out on some neat surprises. Later, as a codependent person, I tried to take on my friend's challenges, but that kept her in a state of unhealthy dependence. It's natural to allow ourselves to be carried, especially when we're having a difficult time, and it's no picnic being broke or bipolar. Being carried doesn't make for a happy life, though. God wants to guide us into wiser thinking and larger capabilities. For that, we must stand up and go where He leads.

In addition to helping people wisely, Jesus took care of Himself by creating lifestyle boundaries. Although He ministered to thousands, He only traveled with twelve, and He made sure to get alone time with the Father.

I am no Jesus, but if He's my example, I must mimic not only His compassion but His healthy sense of boundaries. Without both, I'll burn out and hurt those I want to help.

If like me, you're learning how to love as Jesus did, today's verse may change your life. Decide in your heart how much to give and don't just respond to pressure or guilt. When you live with healthy boundaries, you'll find you enjoy giving your time, friendships, and resources without resentment. You will feel rich and have enough energy left to spread God's love generously wherever you go.

Sometimes, it becomes necessary to love people from a distance. It's okay to walk away and trust God to take care of someone who is:

- Abusing or controlling you.
- Helping you remain in bondage to a destructive habit.
- Making it hard for you to remain Christ-like.

Jesus came to set you free.

If you need help learning how to keep friendships without losing yourself, I highly recommend *Boundaries* by Dr. Henry Cloud and Dr. John Townsend. It saved my sanity and a long-term friendship for which I'm grateful.

Pray.

Lord, thank You for loving me and giving more than I could ever repay. I am overwhelmed with Your generosity. Examine my relationships, please. Is there anywhere I am not being responsible? Is there anywhere I'm preventing someone else from learning responsibility? If so, please forgive me. Teach me to do my part and remind me that I'm only one of many resources You will use in the lives of those around me.

Think.

Have you been feeling resentful or panicky lately? Sometimes these feelings come when we don't understand the role we play, or when others fail to meet our expectations. God expects us to help one another, but each of us is responsible for the life He's given us.

Act.

Ask God to give you grace, and then talk to the person involved. Remember that God is the source of all you need. Open up to His solutions. You may be surprised.

Day 20: The One Who Sees Me

by Pastor Jimmy John Sill

A good father's love is protective, complete, wholesome, inviting, and warm. Restoration from all hurt, all discomfort, all doubt can be found in the true love of a father. Our Heavenly Father's love is just that– vast, unending, infinite, inexhaustible.

You can be both His beautiful, magnificent, wonderful masterpiece and also an enormous fixer-upper at the same time. You are worth more than silver, more precious than gold to Him. No matter what has happened, or is still happening, or may continue to happen in your life, God sees you and loves you through it all. He is the God who sees. "El Roi" is Hebrew for "The God of Omnipotence and Omnipresence." He revealed himself this way to Hagar, a runaway slave in a desperate situation who felt as if her whole world was a lie.

Genesis 16:13 ESV

So she called the name of the Lord who spoke to her, "You are a God of seeing," for she said, "Truly here I have seen him who looks after me."

Maybe the adversary keeps planting doubts in your head about who you are:

- Who could trust you? A liar when convenient, coming from a complicated past. You cheated in your last relationship, on your last exam; you lied to your best friend because you couldn't deal with their drama today. You called into work because you stayed out too late. #liar-liar

- Who could want you? In doubt of your beauty, your worth. Envious of honest success. You're a single teenage parent who's striving to provide and depending on others. Your friends have finished college and have good jobs and great relationships. #alone

- Who could love you? Shame and guilt cover you, eating you up from the inside out. The burden of humiliation and remorse are unbearable at times; you consider a dark path. #nowayout

STOP.

Let's agree that Satan, whom Revelations 12:10 calls the Accuser, wants to darken our image of God and diminish His character within us. He tells us we will always be the same sinful, regretful, and condemned self. He wants us to forget the truths that:

- God is ever-present – inescapable. #always
- God sees through you – penetrating. #adored
- God loves you always – boundless. #forever

We cannot escape God's pursuit. He knows what we desire and what we think about. As we sleep, as we wake, as we do our day-to-day things, God is there. God asked His own Son to die so you would not have to. Our Father's love is so vast and His mercy so boundless that Jesus willingly paid your debt and the debt of all the people of the world. #Immeasurablelove!

Psalm 139:1-18 ESV

[1]O Lord, you have searched me and known me! [2]You know when I sit down and when I rise up; You discern my thoughts from afar. [3]You search out my path and my lying down and are acquainted with all my ways. [4]Even before a word is on my tongue, behold, O Lord, you know it altogether.

[5]You hem me in, behind and before, and lay your hand upon me. [6]Such knowledge is too wonderful for me; it is high; I cannot attain it. [7]Where shall I go from your Spirit? Or where shall I flee from your presence?

[8]If I ascend to heaven, you are there! If I make my bed in Sheol[3], you are there! [9]If I take the wings of the morning and dwell in the uttermost parts of the sea, [10]even there your hand shall lead me, and your right hand shall hold me.

[11]If I say, "Surely the darkness shall cover me, and the light about me be night," [12]even the darkness is not dark to you; the night is bright as the day, for darkness is as light with you.

[13]For you formed my inward parts; you knitted me together in my mother's womb. [14]I praise you, for I am fearfully and wonderfully made. Wonderful are your works; my soul knows it very well.

[15]My frame was not hidden from you when I was being made in secret, intricately woven in the depths of the earth. [16]Your eyes saw my unformed substance; in your book were written, every one of them, the days that were formed for me, when as yet there was none of them.

---

[3] Sheol: The place of the dead. Link for more info:
https://www.gotquestions.org/sheol-hades-hell.html

[17] How precious to me are your thoughts, O God! How vast is the sum of them! [18] If I would count them, they are more than the sand. I awake, and I am still with you.

I am worthy, I am pure, I am successful, I am not alone, I am loved. How we long for reinforcement on all these terms. Everyone wants to know that they are worth the investment of time and relationship. We all desire success, wanting kudos for a job "Well Done." We also want to know that we are not alone in our pursuits.

In John 8:1-11 NLT, the Pharisees marched a woman up to Jesus, in front of a crowd. [4]"Teacher," they said to Jesus, "this woman was caught in the act of adultery. [5] The law of Moses says to stone her. What do you say?"

Jesus replied, [7]"All right, but let the one who has never sinned throw the first stone!" One by one, they left and Jesus said to her, [10b] "Didn't even one of them condemn you?"

[11]"No, Lord," she said.

And Jesus said, "Neither do I. Go and sin no more."

This woman had given herself to a false love and was left alone to face a death penalty. True love gives restoration, honor, and life to all who accept it. Look up into the Father's eyes and gain acceptance of who you really are. Go and live a life of freedom and be a testimony to the unfathomable love of Jesus Christ!

Pray.

You know me, You knit me, You see me, yet You desire to be with me. Thank You for Your persistent, all-consuming love. Father, I love that You that relentlessly pursued me. You never took Your watchful eyes off me. You delivered me from so many hurtful situations. In the times You could not keep me from harm because of my stubbornness, Your heart broke, but You never stopped loving me.

Forgive me for those times. Restore me and renew me as I pursue You. Let us together revel in the joy that is Your presence. Grant me peace and strength as my days continue, until I come home to see You face to face. In Jesus's Name, amen.

Think.

Meditate on "The One Who Sees You" this week. Write down what God has delivered you from, not to glorify your past, but to memorialize God's pursuit of you.

Maybe you struggle with doubt and uncertainty, thinking, "God can't deliver me from _____."

God is more than enough.

He is faithful and will set you back on straight street, giving you power to overcome and help others with the same struggles.

Act.

Write down a verse from today's lesson and carry it with you. When the devil accuses you, whether true or false, pull out that verse and look up to the One Who Sees You and loves you.

Day 21: Embracing Self-Love

by: Debra Trappen

Psalm 139 TPT

*[14]I thank you, God, for making me so mysteriously complex!
Everything you do is marvelously breathtaking. It simply
amazes me to think about it! How thoroughly you know me,
Lord! [15]You even formed every bone in my body when you
created me in the secret place, carefully, skillfully shaping me
from nothing to something.*

Ephesians 2:10 NLT

*For we are God's masterpiece. He has created us anew in
Christ Jesus, so we can do the good things he planned for us
long ago.*

1 Thessalonians 1:4 TPT

*Dear brothers and sisters, you are dearly loved by God and we
know that he has chosen you to be his very own.*

Before we dig into this message together, I want to share
some shocking statistics:

- Only 4% of women around the world consider
  themselves beautiful.[4]

---

[4] https://www.dove.com/us/en/stories/about-dove/our-research.html.

- 80% of women agree that every woman has something about her that is beautiful but do not see their own beauty. [4]

- 63% of men always feel like they could lose some weight, but 65% of them are willing to date someone who is overweight. [5]

- 38% of men would give a year of their life for a "perfect body." [6]

My darling, you are a masterpiece. You are divinely beautiful, truly fearfully and wonderfully made. You were created to be UNIQUE and are so loved by God. It is time to embrace self-love. My heart's desire is for you to embrace these truths, not the lies of unrealistic perfection this world wants you to believe.

I was raised in the Lutheran Church. I knew Jesus and all the songs that told me He loved me. When I was ten, someone told me I was beautiful BUT chubby. I let those thoughts in, and they stayed deep inside me. "Being chubby" meant so many things to me. I couldn't wear those tiny clothes in the movies, magazine ads, and my favorite TV shows. That was when my negative self-talk about my body began and my internal dialogue became toxic.

My inner voice said, "You're ugly; you're fat; no one wants a chubby friend." It cut more deeply with thoughts like, "You know that boy moved because you take up too much

[5] Bryann Mannino, "TODAY/AOL 'Ideal to Real' body image survey results," Feb. 24, 2014.
https://www.aol.com/article/2014/02/24/loveyourselfie/20836450/.

[6] "Reflections on Body Image: All Party Parliamentary Group on Body Image," YMCA: http://ymca-central-assets.s3-eu-west-1.amazonaws.com/s3fs-public/APPG-Reflections-on-body-image.pdf.

space… why can't you be smaller?" I would get the lead in a school play and think, "I only got it because they feel sorry for me since I'm chubby." I discounted my God-given talents all the time.

The image in the mirror and the number on the scale became my obsessions. In seventh grade, I taped a poster of workout moves on the back of my door. I did each exercise so many times I would lose count. As I grew taller, my body slimmed, but that didn't take my thoughts off my body. My mind space was filled with how I looked and what outfit I wore. By the time I was a freshman in college, I was a size 4-6; yet, my self-talk was evil as ever. I was devastated and angry. All that hard work didn't make me feel better or happier. I felt worse.

I turned to the world for comfort, not God. It wasn't pretty. I looked to people to tell me my worth. When I didn't get what I needed, my self-talk would kick in and tell me I wasn't worthy of love, or friendship, or success.

I would pray about it, but I never actually gave the pain and negative thoughts to God. If I did, I'd promptly snatch them back as I was getting ready and looking in the mirror. Sadly, I became a CEO at church (a Christmas and Easter Only attendee). I was lost.

In my mid-20's, I met my husband. Looks don't make a romance. Laughter and connection do. I finally realized I could be loved for something other than what I looked like. It was a dream, an answered prayer.

When we started going to church together, I was reminded of who GOD tells me I am and whose I am. Daily time with God went from five minutes of hurried prayer to an hour abiding with Him in the morning. I packed my playlists with affirming worship songs and listened to evening meditations on

Scripture. Ultimately, my negative self-talk was replaced with what God thinks of me. The healing began.

A few months ago, I was doing Yoga in the dim light of my studio. My guide was whispering sweet instructions: hold, stretch, breeeeeathe… In that moment I realized I was talking to myself again. This time, my words were sweet, kind, and encouraging. I was thanking my body for never giving up on me during the years I was so cruel to her. I was promising to love and nurture her until the end.

My darling, trust God when He says you are HIS chosen one. He loves you and will redeem every moment you've lost to negative self-talk. Today, God is using me to speak to hundreds of thousands of women. Each week, I empower and inspire them to define and design the best version of themselves. As they ditch the senseless hustle for worldly perfection, they live out loud and divinely on purpose!

He has a plan for you, too. Abide with Him every single day, and He will bless you with wisdom and vision beyond your wildest dreams.

XXOO

Pray.

Magnificent Heavenly Father!

In this moment, I am longing to embrace honor and love my body.

I believe You, when You tell me I am fearfully and wonderfully made; yet, my self-love struggle remains. Your divine word reminds me that my happiness, joy, and worth come from You - not the number on a scale or a size tag.

My deepest desire is to refocus my thoughts and energy on You, Father. As I abide with You more, I am trusting You will take care of everything else.

Create in me a clean heart. Fill it with love, peace, and forgiveness…Grant me the blissful ability to see myself as You see me.

Think.

It's time to write custom affirmations!

1. Start by writing out the negative things you say to yourself. They may flow all at once, or they may take a few days to come out. Please give yourself extra grace as you complete this step. It can be shocking when you see the words written out in black and white.

2. On a fresh page, take each one of those thoughts and FLIP THEM. Turn the negative thoughts into an affirming statement about whatever you're focusing on and be specific. These will become the foundation of your custom affirmations, so consider starting these statements with "I am" or "God says I am!"

3. Find one Scripture to support each statement and complete each divine affirmation!

This exercise will help you shine a light on the lies you tell yourself. It will also help you replace those thoughts with divinely inspired words.

Act.

1. Print out your affirmations. Place them where you will see them every single day: on your bathroom mirror, in your phone as a calendar item or the lock screen, inside your journal, on your refrigerator—you get the idea.

2. Write yourself love notes. Grab a pad of sticky notes and start writing out quick words of encouragement to yourself. Focus on those areas you wrote down that tend to bring negative thoughts. Be sure to include congratulation notes for successes. Write about areas where you excel!

    Spread these throughout your space. Put notes in your car, inside your handbag/backpack, on your mirrors, at the front door, inside your pantry, where you grab your coffee/tea mugs, and so on!

3. Encourage someone else to join you on this journey of self-love. Share your affirmation exercise with your best friend or someone you are mentoring. Earlier, I shared statistics that confirm almost everyone in your world feels insecure. Conquer this together. Your self-love bestie will become your go-to person, someone you can talk to in those darker moments along the way. Celebrate together when you conquer the negative voices in your mind!

4. Make a playlist. Here are some songs I use to support my self-love mindset:

    "Who You Say I Am" – Hillsong

    "You Say" – Lauren Daigel

    "Beautifully Broken" – Plumb

Week 4: Your Sea Legs are Getting Stronger.

Day 22: Competitive

by Kristi Bridges

Ecclesiastes 4 NLT

[7] *I observed yet another example of something meaningless under the sun.* [8] *This is the case of a man who is all alone, without a child or a brother, yet who works hard to gain as much wealth as he can. But then he asks himself, "Who am I working for? Why am I giving up so much pleasure now?" It is all so meaningless and depressing.*

[9] *Two people are better off than one, for they can help each other succeed.* [10] *If one person falls, the other can reach out and help. But someone who falls alone is in real trouble.* [11] *Likewise, two people lying close together can keep each other warm. But how can one be warm alone?* [12] *A person standing alone can be attacked and defeated, but two can stand back-to-back and conquer. Three are even better, for a triple-braided cord is not easily broken.*

I took a personality test once and laughed as I shared the results with my coworker, Stacy. "Most of the results were exactly right, but can you believe they called me competitive? Cray-cray."

"I can see that," Stacy said. I was stunned. Maybe she thought I said, "Collaborative." Nope. No static on our line—she had heard me correctly. I like to think of myself as generous, compassionate, supportive. I hate competing because I don't want to make anyone feel bad.

Stacy has a master's degree in leadership development, and she understands me as though we were twins. Still, I tried to argue my way out of this one. I finally admitted that yes, maybe I compete with myself at times. She gracefully moved on to other topics.

Ever since that conversation, I've noticed signs Stacy and the personality test may have been right. "Competitive" sounds uncharitable. I believe everyone should explore their own potential and make the world a colorful place. Yet the other day, I found myself watching a speaker and feeling not only competitive but jealous. "I could do that," I thought. I had wanted that spot.

Shocked? Nice people aren't supposed to admit to such feelings, but they turn toxic if we don't. On the way home, I talked to God about it. *What's at the root of this? Why do I feel frustrated? I know You're at work in both our lives. Why didn't I just enjoy her message? I don't even remember the message. Fix me please, Lord.*

Ever since I was a kid, I've watched others do interesting things and said, "I could do that!" This desire for equivalent coolness has spurred me to improve my poetry, learn guitar, ride my bike with no hands, and develop other skills which have made life an adventure. It's led me to shoot for the stars more than once. My co-trainer and I have the best kind of friendly competition. Each of us is determined not to let the other take on a bigger workload. When things get off-balance, we invent things to do. We care about each other, but we also want to prove ourselves.

Here's a paraphrase of the Oxford Dictionary's definition of Competitiveness [7] : desiring to be more successful than

---

[7] *English Oxford Living Dictionaries* online, "Competitiveness," https://en.oxforddictionaries.com/definition/competitiveness.

others, be as good or better than others, or compare well in terms of pricing (perceived value). Learning to do what others can do makes me feel smart.

My co-trainer and I like to compare well in terms of our accomplishments. At the end of the day, we must earn our keep.

It turns out thirteen of the sixteen Myers-Briggs Personality Types have a competitive side. Some people compete with others, some compete with themselves, always seeking to do better than before. It keeps us fresh. Life is long and atrophy awaits those who stop trying.

Why did I refuse to see myself this way? I saw competition as something that hurts people. Do you know someone who takes competition to extremes? They take joy in crushing you. They make snide comments, use sabotage, or attempt to control resources as though there's not enough. That behavior drives away true happiness. Some coaches, instead of inspiring us to greatness, call us inadequate if we're not conquering everyone else. Insecurity is a strong motivator, but it can cause anxiety and dysfunction in our relationships.

Where's the line? Whether you compete against your own past successes or find a friendly coworker to keep you on your toes, keep these things in mind:

What is the benefit? If you're feeling competitive or being challenged, consider what you could gain. Better skills, recognition, the chance to develop panache under pressure?

Are you using a single activity to judge an entire person? Maintain compassion. A friend told me she sometimes leaves our group of friends feeling like a failure. I've felt that way, too. Our people are positive, creative, and motivated. At times, I feel I can't keep up. When she voiced her feelings, we discussed it as a group. Bottom line—nobody's judging us. We each have our own path and pace. We were making self-judgments, and they were demotivating and unhelpful. Left unchecked, these feelings could have destroyed our friendship with those whose only crime was enthusiasm.

Is it competition or jealousy? Competition can make you a winner, even if someone else reaches the goal first. Any time you stretch for a new distance, you benefit. Jealousy slows you down. When we're jealous, the negative energy drags on us and absorbs the attention we should spend on enjoyable, productive activities. Nobody wants to be around a jealous person.

Are you operating with a lack mindset? God created a universe that is still expanding. He has a plan for your life, and it includes wonderful things, people, and experiences which will work together to create a whole package. If you're worried about not winning the soulmate you want, landing the job you want, or getting the last perfect apartment, let it go.

Psalm 37 NLT

³ Trust in the LORD and do good.
Then you will live safely in the land and prosper.

⁴ Take delight in the LORD, and he
will give you your heart's desires.

Pray.

Lord, help me to trust You and do my best. I'll celebrate the accomplishments of those around me without measuring myself by them, and I'll look for ways to partner with people, because two or three are better than one alone.

Think.

Are you having trouble with jealousy or feelings of inadequacy? Have you noticed that people are tense around you?

Act.

Walk yourself through the questions above. Talk to someone who will share honest observations with you. And pray—God has a plan for the person who's in the place you want, and He has a plan for you as well. Our Creator doesn't short anyone who's willing to follow His lead.

Day 23: Headwinds v Tailwinds

by Kristi Bridges

2 Kings 6 NLT

¹⁵ *When the servant of the man of God got up early the next morning and went outside, there were troops, horses, and chariots everywhere. "Oh, sir, what will we do now?" the young man cried to Elisha.*

¹⁶ *"Don't be afraid!" Elisha told him. "For there are more on our side than on theirs!"* ¹⁷ *Then Elisha prayed, "O LORD, open his eyes and let him see!" The LORD opened the young man's eyes, and when he looked up, he saw that the hillside around Elisha was filled with horses and chariots of fire.*

Imagine you're on a bicycle in Colorado. The day is perfect. You bought a new bottle with the filter inside, so you can refill it in a cold mountain stream. Your backpack is a party with a zipper, carrying lunch, your awesome new camera, rain gear, and sunscreen. You pass someone with no backpack and give yourself a thumbs-up. You Super Scout, you! Your legs feel strong, and you pedal harder just because you can.

You're grateful for the time off work. Your boss was impressed at your vacation plans, but you discounted it by saying, "Well, I haven't trained as hard as I could have."

That's called self-handicapping. Before we try something, we come up with reasons we might fail. It's an attempt to save face, just in case. It's a comfort move you need to lose. To your boss—an achiever—self-handicapping is like going on stage with a pacifier.

"TMBWAHNTBWA!"

"What's Hamlet saying?"

For a better impression, say, "Thank you! I'm excited." Confidence is attractive.

As you pedal, thoughts of work buzz at the rhythm of your strokes. Your boss gets on your nerves. How did she get that job anyway? Some people can charm their way into anything.

Whoo, this uphill thing is tough. You hear water around the bend and push work out of your mind. Immediately, you notice the cool breeze on your sweaty skin. The twitter of birds rings a musical telegraph along the mountain.

You stretch, and the packless cyclist pedals by. He waves cheerfully and suddenly your pack weighs fifty pounds. You set it down and fill your bottle in the stream. As you drink, you think of the cheery, packless cyclist. "That guy probably works out every day. Some of us don't have that kind of time."

You consider lightening your pack. The sun is out—if you leave your rain gear behind that bush, it's not exactly littering. You're just leaving something behind for someone who might need it.

You only think about it. You're not actually a litterbug.

You hoist your pack and get on the bike. Three miles to the top. You told people you might not make it. Self-handicapping makes quitting easier. You're not a quitter, though. Even if you don't win, you go all the way. That's the kind of person you are.

What kind of person are you? Adventurous! Prepared! A Finisher! James Clear[8] says, "Each action you take is a vote for

---

[8] James Clear, *Atomic Habits: An Easy & Proven Way to Build God Habits & Break Bad Ones (Avery: New York, 2018)*.

the type of person that you believe that you are." Vote with your feet!

The last half mile is a doozy, but you rock it. When you reach the peak, you celebrate with a little lunch. Squirrels like Fritos®, so you share. King of the World, that's you. The real king comes out of the woods; you freeze. You've seen minivans smaller than that bear. You hoist your pack and jump on your bike. It's a downhill ride—your legs needed a break. Sunset is coming—you needed to get back. These things don't cheer a mind filled with fur and claws.

We naturally give more attention to our challenges or "headwinds," than the ways in which we're being helped. When you're escaping the bear who wants to share, you're unlikely to give thanks for the downhill slope and boost in speed. They simply don't feel important.

This is called The Headwinds/ Tailwinds Asymmetry. We focus on obstacles to overcome. Unchecked, this can become a joy-blocker. We meet metaphorical bears every day, but when they fill our heads, we don't appreciate our tailwinds. If instead, we take note of events and people that make life easier, we're happier.

Our future gets brighter as well. How is that possible?

You work hard, so when someone else sits in the boss's chair, you assume she was lucky. What if, instead of being resentful, you make her job easier, and she teaches you things she's learned from previous positions? You'll become more marketable and enjoy work more.

You came to the mountain prepared, so when someone whizzes by you, you identify all the ways you have it tough. Shai Davidai and Tom Gilovich, who researched the

Headwinds/Tailwinds Asymmetry[9] found that nearly everyone assumes they have it harder than other people. In nearly every sibling pair they interviewed, each claimed to have had the tougher childhood. Do you know the other cyclist's story? Quit judging. Would you have been happier with no lunch?

Think of resentment as an off-switch to gratitude. When the light is off, it's easier to trip. People who feel things are unjust are more likely to be unhappy and make moral compromises. That explains the temptation to be a litterbug. Thank goodness you'd never do that.

Warning: Don't tell someone, "You have so much to be grateful for!" God sprinkles every day with delights, but people bristle when we accuse them of being ungrateful. Just model gratitude. They'll catch on.

Pray.

Thank You, Lord! You protect me in ways I don't even know, and You give me reasons to enjoy each day. Bless those who have helped me. I'll choose to be alert and appreciative.

Think.

What talents, skills, and people do you have on your side?

---

[9] Davidai S, Gilovich T., "The headwinds/tailwinds asymmetry: An availability bias in assessments of barriers and blessings," The National Center for Biotechnology Information, Dec 2016, https://www.ncbi.nlm.nih.gov/pubmed/27869473.

Act.

For the rest of this month, end the day by journaling thanks for three things:

1. Someone who helped you.
2. Something which inspired you or made you smile.
3. Something you accomplished.

Day 24: Riot or Rescue

by Richard Staley, PhD.

Acts 19 NLT

[23] About that time, serious trouble developed in Ephesus concerning the Way. [24] It began with Demetrius, a silversmith who had a large business manufacturing silver shrines of the Greek goddess Artemis.[e] He kept many craftsmen busy. [25] He called them together, along with others employed in similar trades, and addressed them as follows:

"Gentlemen, you know that our wealth comes from this business. [26] But as you have seen and heard, this man Paul has persuaded many people that handmade gods aren't really gods at all…"

[28] At this their anger boiled, and they began shouting, "Great is Artemis of the Ephesians!" [29] Soon the whole city was filled with confusion. Everyone rushed to the amphitheater, dragging along Gaius and Aristarchus, who were Paul's traveling companions from Macedonia. [30] Paul wanted to go in, too, but the believers wouldn't let him. [31] Some of the officials of the province, friends of Paul, also sent a message to him, begging him not to risk his life by entering the amphitheater.

In this passage, there was a riot taking place in the city of Ephesus. Demetrius, the silversmith, had stirred up the people. He'd convinced other silversmiths their trade was in jeopardy, and they would lose their livelihoods. Paul was determined to go into the theater, which held approximately 25,000 people, and try to rescue his traveling companions. His disciples would not allow him to do so. Even his non-believing friends in the government convinced him that entering the melee was a bad idea. This could have resulted in physical harm or even premature death for Paul.

Have you ever been on the verge of something that could have been harmful, and your friends or family—or even strangers—stopped you from making a bad decision? Maybe you were the one who prevented a friend or family member from doing something harmful. An act of intervention may not always be appreciated at the time, but when you have time to think and reflect on things, you see the wisdom of those who intervened.

Paul was typically led by the Spirit, always checking with the Lord to find out what action he should take. In this situation, he appears to have acted more impulsively. The Lord used his disciples and even non-believing friends to spare him from harm.

Someone once spared me from making an ill-advised decision that would have certainly resulted in harm. I grew up going to church and was saved at an early age, but I had a season when I stopped going to church and was not serving the Lord. I was in a night club one evening, and someone else had a ball cap I picked up and put on. Wearing hats in this particular establishment was not permitted. One of the gentlemen hired by the club to maintain order—of which there were several—approached me and politely requested that I remove the hat. I was involved in competitive weight lifting and thought I could take care of myself in most situations. To put it simply, I was acting the fool. I resisted the request and started stating my case, which was not well thought out. Suddenly, a young lady at my table grabbed the hat, threw it on the floor, and said, "Shut up." That seemed to satisfy the gentleman in charge, and he left the table. Then the young lady said, "They will take you outside and make an example out of you." I quickly reflected on the situation and concluded that she was right and kept me from certain danger.

Reflect on your past and give the Lord thanks for the times He used others to keep you from making a poor decision, or even being injured, or worse. 1 Corinthians 15:57 KJV says, "But thanks be to God, which giveth us the victory through our Lord Jesus Christ." Some translations substitute "who" for "which," but I believe "which" is correct, because it is giving thanks that brings the victory.

Pray.

Father, in the precious name of Jesus my Lord, I thank You for all the times that You have intervened on my behalf to keep me from making a bad decision or getting into a harmful situation. Thank You for the people You have used to help me—whether family, friends, or strangers. And thank You Lord, for the times You have used me to prevent someone from danger. I desire to be more sensitive to Your Spirit to lead, guide, and correct me in my daily living. In Jesus's name, amen.

Think.

1. Have you taken time recently to thank the Lord for people that He has put in your life to help you make good decisions?

2. What can you do to become more sensitive to the Holy Spirit as He guides and corrects you on a daily basis?

3. Have you asked the Lord to use you to minister to others—family, friends, or even strangers?

4. Have you made yourself available to do that?

Act.

Set a lunchtime reminder on your calendar to pray and connect with the Holy Spirit. Ask God to lead you and thank Him for the friends and family He's given you.

Day 25: Truth Pact - Part 1

by Kristi Bridges

Acts 24: 16 ESV

So I always take pains to have a clear conscience toward both God and man.

"Who dumped all the fish food in the tank?" my stepdad demanded.

"I don't know," I replied. There were two adults and one seven-year-old in the house—me. Who do you think did it?

"You'll get in less trouble if you just tell the truth," Mom said. I didn't buy it.

Growing up, I frequently shouted, "You never believe me!" to which Mom would reply, "Give me a reason!" With practice, I got better at lying and even better at hiding my actions, so I didn't have to lie. Then one day when I was 22, I found myself bawling in front of the office manager at work.

I'd had a busy weekend, so Monday I called in sick, sounding as miserable as I could. I felt miraculously better the moment I hung up. I made myself breakfast and sat down to read my Bible.

Proverbs 12:22 ESV

<u>Lying lips</u> are an abomination to the LORD, but those who act faithfully are his delight.

Eek. I flipped a few pages.

Proverbs 6:16-20 ESV

There are six things that the LORD hates, seven that are an abomination to him: haughty eyes, <u>a lying tongue</u>, and hands that shed innocent blood, a heart that devises wicked plans, feet that make haste to run to evil, a false witness who breathes out lies, and one who sows discord among brothers. My son, keep your father's commandment, and forsake not your mother's teaching.

My stomach hurt. Lord, are you trying to make me sick?

Revelation 21: 8 ESV

But as for the cowardly, the faithless, the detestable, as for murderers, the sexually immoral, sorcerers, idolaters, and <u>all liars</u>, their portion will be in the lake that burns with fire and sulfur, which is the second death.

Good grief. Cowardly liars in line with murderers. But Lord, I just wanted some time with You—that's not so bad, right?

Psalm 24 ESV

³ Who shall ascend the hill of the LORD? And who shall stand in his holy place? ⁴ He who has clean hands and a pure heart, who does not lift up his soul to what is false and does not swear <u>deceitfully</u>. ⁵ He will receive blessing from the LORD and righteousness from the God of his salvation.

Jesus came to give us abundant life and an intimate, powerful relationship with our Creator. This kind of life comes from doing things God's way, even when we've only had three hours sleep and could use a day off.

By 10 a.m., I sat in Teresa's office tearfully confessing. She wrinkled her face like I was a loon. "It's okay, everybody calls in. What do you want to do?" I offered to work the rest of the day.

In Luke 16 ESV, Jesus said, "[10]One who is faithful in a very little is also faithful in much, and one who is dishonest in a very little is also dishonest in much. [11]If then you have not been faithful in the unrighteous wealth, who will entrust to you the true riches? [12]And if you have not been faithful in that which is another's, who will give you that which is your own?"

Our potential increases as we face the challenges of righteous living. When I stopped saying, "(cough, cough,) I'm sick today," I learned to balance my time more wisely. Now I'm not exhausted Monday morning when the people paying my bills expect me to do my job. If I'm bored at work, I develop skills in areas which interest me. Sometimes I simply set a timer and say, "Thank You, Lord, for this paycheck. I'm gonna knock out this boring task in fifty minutes."

Once I decided to stop lying, I realized our shop director was a liar as well. When a client would call with a rush request, he would make promises he couldn't keep. "Sure, I'll have that part shipped out tomorrow." Three days later, I'd answer the phone to an angry customer with no part. This lost us a lot of business. Instead of being a yes-man, a wise shop director would have been honest. "That sounds distressing. It will take three days for us to get that part together, but we'll ship it as soon as it's ready." Our clients might have called someone else in a pinch, but they would have continued to trust us.

Was he really lying? It's possible he didn't know how long things took to build, even though he'd been the boss for over a year. In any case, a client feels deceived when a promise is unfulfilled.

Proverbs 20:25 NIV says, "It is a trap to dedicate something rashly and only later to consider one's vows." It's wiser to follow the rule, "Under-promise and over-deliver." Say, "I'll get back to you," instead of "Yes." No matter how pressured you feel or how much you want to do something, don't agree until you have reviewed your schedule, your budget, and your personal need for rest.

I've missed a deadline and had to confess I was unprepared. That's embarrassing, and I certainly don't want to have those conversations often. However, when I don't cover my mistakes with excuses, my reputation as a woman of integrity grows and so do my opportunities.

Pray.

Lord, I realize truth matters to You. I hate to lose face with people, and I'm not a fan of conflict. It's easier to lie or fudge the truth, but I don't want what's easy. I want what You have for me. Forgive me please and help me to be a person of integrity. In Jesus's name, amen.

Think.

When are you most tempted to deceive or make excuses? How can you adjust your life to avoid doing wrong?

Act.

Who have you deceived? Pray first, and then talk to that person. Apologize and let them know you are determined to be honest from now on. Be careful not to promise anything you won't do.

Day 26: Truth Pact - Part 2

by Kristi Bridges

Colossians 3:9-10 ESV

Do not lie to one another, seeing that you have put off the old self with its practices and have put on the new self, which is being renewed in knowledge after the image of its creator.

Ephesians 4:15 ESV

Rather, speaking the truth in love, we are to grow up in every way into him who is the head, into Christ...

Yesterday, we talked about being truthful at work and following through on commitments. Today, let's explore two areas where deception is even more tempting – personal relationships and self-talk.

Ephesians tells us to speak the truth in love. In a world of networking and surface conversations, we need friends who will be real with us. I bet you would never say, "You look terrific!" when there's toilet paper hanging from someone's pants. Is it just as easy to speak up when you might hurt their feelings?

Let's say your friend Bob asks to borrow money, but he hasn't paid you back for your prior loans. If you're tired of funding Bottomless Bob, you might start avoiding him, letting the friendship fade away. If you care about your friendship, you may feel guilty about refusing to help him out. Resentment could build until one day you're shouting, "Am I Bob's Bank? Get a job, Bob!" Ouch.

What if you prayed first, and then said, "No. I get resentful when you borrow money and don't pay it back." It's possible Bob has lost other friends who weren't kind enough to speak up.

Be prepared to deal with emotions. Bob may feel helpless and desperate. God can help him work his way into a better financial state. Let him know you care and want to be his friend. If mooching is a lifestyle for Bob, you may never see him again. However, if he cares about the friendship, it will become stronger because he knows he can trust you to be straightforward.

Once you've expressed your feelings, avoid nagging. When we believe someone is doing things wrong, we try to parent them. That's destructive. If Bob asks for advice on budgeting, have one conversation, and then let Bob handle things. Continue to refuse loans without nagging, "Got my cash?"

It takes practice. Everyone communicates differently. When I have trouble talking to someone gracefully, I send an email or text. Whenever I pray first, things turn out much better. I pray, "Lord, help me to say only what You would have me say—no more and no less. Please begin softening this person's heart even before I send this, so they'll receive what I'm trying to say." Afterwards, I try to restrain myself from sending an onslaught of further explanations, because the more I talk, the messier things get. I'm not always successful, but God gives grace.

How well do you accept this kind of honesty? You spent eighteen years being corrected. The last four years or more, you fought for self-esteem when faced with bullies and betrayal. You're finally grown-up and on your own, for the most part. When someone gives you feedback, you might get defensive. Plus, they may be misunderstanding you. Pray before responding. Consider how your actions have been perceived and ask God to help you give this person His love.

Psalm 51:6 ESV

Behold, you delight in truth in the inward being, and you teach me wisdom in the secret heart.

I John 1:6 ESV

If we say we have fellowship with him while we walk in darkness, we lie and do not practice the truth.

Are you honest with yourself? Many of us have an inner voice that's overly critical and a silencer who says, "I'm fine, turn up the music." Neither of these voices is completely honest. You are beautiful. God made you unique and interesting and talented.

You are also wearing a body filled with hormones and hunger and a brain that sometimes goes to extremes. As long as you're in that body, you'll make mistakes and hopefully, you'll work to resist temptation. The better you are at being honest with yourself, the happier you will be.

Follow God's example. When God confronted me about lying, He didn't gloss over it. He didn't say, "It's so sweet that you want to spend time with Me, so I'm going to ignore it." Our loving Father is not interested in spoiling us, so we'll feel loved. That kind of love has a tolerance-building effect, like pot or opioids. When a parent withholds correction in an effort to be loving, children become more selfish. They grow up to be miserable adults, because they didn't develop the character needed for satisfying relationships.

The Lord tells us clearly which behavior is righteous and which is sinful, so we can choose the best life possible. He lets us experience the consequences of our actions, so we make better choices. At the same time, He gave us an unimaginable sacrifice through Christ when we least deserved it, to let us know nothing could ever separate us from His love.

When your inner critic calls you hopeless, say, "God doesn't think so." When you've sinned or behaved unwisely, confess and say, "Lord, I'm sorry." Then make the change ASAP, so you don't get into the rut of rationalization.

Pray.

Lord, thank You for loving me more than I could ever deserve and for giving me clear direction. Help me respond gracefully to feedback and speak the truth in love.

Think.

Is there someone who's getting on your nerves? Have you been truthful with that person? How could you behave differently in this relationship?

Act.

Make a truth pact with yourself. From this point forward, decide to tell the truth every time. Then check out the song, "If We're Honest," by Francesca Battistelli.

Day 27: Lead

by Kristi Bridges

1 Kings 3 NLT

*³ Solomon loved the L*ORD *and followed all the decrees of his father, David, except that Solomon, too, offered sacrifices and burned incense at the local places of worship. ⁴ The most important of these places of worship was at Gibeon, so the king went there and sacrificed 1,000 burnt offerings. ⁵ That night the* L*ORD appeared to Solomon in a dream, and God said, "What do you want? Ask, and I will give it to you!"*

⁶ Solomon replied, "You showed great and faithful love to your servant my father, David, because he was honest and true and faithful to you. And you have continued to show this great and faithful love to him today by giving him a son to sit on his throne.

*⁷ "Now, O L*ORD *my God, you have made me king instead of my father, David, but I am like a little child who doesn't know his way around. ⁸ And here I am in the midst of your own chosen people, a nation so great and numerous they cannot be counted! ⁹ Give me an understanding heart so that I can govern your people well and know the difference between right and wrong. For who by himself is able to govern this great people of yours?"*

¹⁰ The Lord was pleased that Solomon had asked for wisdom. ¹¹ So God replied, "Because you have asked for wisdom in governing my people with justice and have not asked for a long life or wealth or the death of your enemies— ¹² I will give you what you asked for! I will give you a wise and understanding heart such as no one else has had or ever will have! ^{13} *And I will also give you what you did not ask for—riches and fame! No other king in all the world will be compared to you for the rest of your life!* ^{14} *And if you follow me and obey my decrees and my commands as your father, David, did, I will give you a long life."*

^{15} *Then Solomon woke up and realized it had been a dream. He returned to Jerusalem and stood before the Ark of the Lord's Covenant, where he sacrificed burnt offerings and peace offerings. Then he invited all his officials to a great banquet.*

Four years before I was eligible to vote, I stood on a corner with a sign, urging adults to vote in my place. The first time I completed my own ballot, my candidate won. I was ecstatic! Two years later, I wanted to slap him for abusing my trust. Voting is too often a choice between bullheaded candidates and those full of manure. Why am I talking politics in the middle of a devotion? I want to vote without vomiting, and I believe you can help.

God has promised to guide you, and I trust Him. Isaiah 30:21 NLT says, "Your own ears will hear him. Right behind you a voice will say, 'This is the way you should go,' whether to the right or to the left."

Somebody reading this book is hearing a call to govern, and I want you to take it seriously. Another reader would rather run off to Antarctica barefoot and gather penguin eggs than run for office. It's okay if politics isn't your calling. Both of you have a part to play.

Solomon knew he needed God's help. In 1 Chronicles 28 ESV, his dad gave him the throne with these words: ^{9}"And you, Solomon my son, know the God of your father and serve him with a whole heart and with a willing mind, for the LORD searches all hearts and understands every plan and thought. If you seek him, he will be found by you, but if you forsake him, he will cast you off forever. [10] Be careful now, for the LORD has chosen you to build a house for the sanctuary; be strong and do it."

Solomon avoided the assignment and gave offerings at the high places. High places were shrines which had been established for violent, sexually destructive, manipulative worship of idols. The Israelites used those same shrines to offer their sacrifices to God, but He wanted them to worship in a place dedicated to holiness, purity, and forgiveness.

Sometimes we procrastinate because we feel overwhelmed or insecure in our abilities. After Solomon saw God, he awoke with power and went to work. His wisdom brought people from all around, and those people brought gifts. He built the temple, engineered water delivery and wrote the book of Proverbs, on which I based my first devotional, *Wisdom— Better than Wishing*.

Proverbs gives great advice:

Proverbs 11 ESV

[14] *Where there is no guidance, a people falls, but in an abundance of counselors there is safety...* [25] *Whoever brings blessing will be enriched, and one who waters will himself be watered.* [26] *The people curse him who holds back grain, but a blessing is on the head of him who sells it.*

Proverbs 21 ESV

[5] *The plans of the diligent lead surely to abundance, but everyone who is hasty comes only to poverty.*

Proverbs 22 ESV

⁷*The rich rules over the poor, and the borrower is the slave of the lender.*

Proverbs 31 ESV

⁸ *Open your mouth for the mute, for the rights of all who are destitute.* ⁹ *Open your mouth, judge righteously, defend the rights of the poor and needy.*

When you see a need for change, do you go to the high places or take action? God will guide you the moment you ask for wisdom. You can trust Him, even when things seem hopeless. Research the issues before you cast your vote, and vote in local elections where it counts the most. Compare the candidates' platforms to the Word of God and look beyond promises to see what candidates have accomplished. Sometimes people use godly causes to get votes with no intention to act on them. Write letters to your representatives and support organizations who work effectively on important matters. James 2:17 NLT says, "So you see, faith by itself isn't enough. Unless it produces good deeds, it is dead and useless."

If you choose to run for office, let me know. I'd love to spread the word.

Pray.

Lord, Solomon was around my age when he became king, but You helped him as long as he walked with You. Thank You for giving me wisdom, too. In what ways can I help You make an impact on our government right now? In what ways can I make a godly impact on society?

Think.

Pick one of the three things you'd most like to change in our world. Imagine you've done it, and you're on a tour in which the guide is describing the impact of this change. Feel the overwhelming gratitude, knowing you and God accomplished this together.

Act.

Think of ways your company or school could offer flexible employment for people with disabilities or ways you could personally serve immigrants, fight human trafficking, or do something else close to God's heart. Email your representatives and join others who are taking action.

Day 28: Fearlessly Facing the Future

by Kristi Bridges, Jimmy John Sills, and Cyndilu Miller

Proverbs 31 NLT

*[25] She is clothed with strength and dignity,
and she laughs without fear of the future.
[26] When she speaks, her words are wise,
and she gives instructions with kindness.*

*[27] She carefully watches everything in her household
and suffers nothing from laziness.*

[28] Her children stand and bless her. Her husband praises her:

*[29] "There are many virtuous and capable women in the world,
but you surpass them all!"*

Proverbs 31 is often thought of as the chick chapter of the Bible, because it's rare to find this many verses in a row written about an excellent woman. However, 2 Timothy 3 NLT says, 16 "All Scripture is inspired by God and is useful to teach us what is true and to make us realize what is wrong in our lives. It corrects us when we are wrong and teaches us to do what is right. [17] God uses it to prepare and equip his people to do every good work."

Sometimes we dismiss good advice because it seems to be written for someone else—someone older, younger, another gender, different. If instead, we pray, "Lord, speak to me through this," we level up in ways we didn't expect. The writers of this book aren't perfect, but we know what it means to laugh fearlessly at the future, because we walk hand in hand with our joyful Creator. Here are a few more letters from our authors.

Dear 18-year-old me,

Do you know how amazing you are? These years have been rocky, but you've come through them laughing and kind. You have some wisdom, but it's going to be put to the test in the next decade. May I give you some advice? Lean on your Father. Not your earthly father, who's a child of God just like you, but on your Heavenly Father.

Trust Him over your feelings, because He has more experience than you. Let Him teach you how to love without losing yourself. He's available but not clingy. He's generous beyond any human capability, but He doesn't compromise His values. He's wise but not controlling. He's not afraid to let people make messes, because that's the only way we learn sometimes. He forgives in advance, knowing we all fall.

Take care of yourself and try not to be Atlas, holding up the world. God uses all of us to do His work, not just Kristi Bridges. Put Him first, live in wisdom, and don't let your shape or your age hold you back. Your power is in your heart and mind, not your looks. And chickie, do you have power!

Eighteen-year-old me, I love you so much. People will be unpredictable, but you're strong, you're eternal, and God is always by your side. Let Him lead you. He won't take you where you think you're going, but He knows your heart better than you do. Psalm 37:4 (NIV) says, "Delight yourself in the Lord, and He will give you the desires of your heart."

Love,
Kristi 2018

~

Dear younger me,

I wanted to let you know as I have entered the second half of life, I was thinking of you earlier today. What would expect me to say if it was half-time, and I could speak to you? I remembered the locker room at half-time – adrenaline, excitement, anxiety, expectation, anticipation as our coach spoke, giving us points which sharpened us, attuned us to be more, to try harder, to dig deeper, to break boundaries and of course beat the other team…

Now that I have your attention, I hope with the same wonder and fear, the coaches of old awakened within us… I will begin.

Look at me… Recognize me… I know you… I know you. I know your hopes and dreams, who, what, and where you wanted to be. I know your fears, the deepest, those from your innermost. I know your hurt… our hurt. I know your shame...our shame. I am not who you thought I would be, I am more…I know freedom. I know salvation. I know mercy and grace. I know acceptance and adoption. I know love without boundaries or conditions… I know where we went to be alone…I felt our loneliness…I saw you making deals... I saw you making empty promises…I saw how you plead with God: Alone, over and over. I also heard His answer to you, again and again.

He is the I AM...Healer, Hope, Father, Friend...You are not forgotten, not forsaken; you are forgiven.

Pastor Jimmy John Sills

~

Hello Cyndi,

Hey there, my name is Cyndilu now. It is thirty-eight years beyond your eighteenth year. I know it's nuts! There were times in 1980 that you wondered if you would survive the year, let alone thirty-eight more years and beyond.

Some of what you will go through, I wish I could keep you from experiencing, but without that, I would not be who I am today. Proverbs 14:12 ESV says, "There is a way that seems right to a man, its end is the way to death." This will become so real to you, and you will cling to the fact that God's love is beyond the power of death!

Proverbs 14:13 ESV says, "Even in laughter the heart may ache, and the end of joy may be grief." This becomes real to you in a way you can't even understand right now, but you know what? You also lean on the understanding that God forgives; God's mercy is new every morning, too!

The night seasons will come, and you will survive them... you will learn to lean on God in ways that carry you through the hardest of hearts and the greatest of fears. You will survive it all. And you will rise again with a voice that is stronger than ever!

There is so much more I would love to share with you, but for now, I am going to simply remind you that YOU are more powerful than you know, and God is listening!

Cyndilu

Pray.

Thank You, Lord, for getting me through times I wondered how—or why—I'd survive. I'm sorry for times I didn't trust You, but I'm so glad I'm following You now. Help me to choose wisely and speak with kindness. I look forward to a future without regrets!

Think.

What would you say to your younger self? Is there anything you'd like to say to us or to another older person in your life?

Act.

Write a letter to your younger self.

You also might want to write a letter to someone who's mentored you or had a good impact on your life. Pray for that person as you send their letter.

Week 5: Enjoy the Journey!

Day 29: The Man of My Dreams

by Sarah Soon

Matthew 22:37 TPT

Jesus answered him, "Love the Lord your God with every passion of your heart, with all the energy of your being, and with every thought that is within you. This is the great and supreme commandment."

Lately, a man in his thirties appears in my dreams. He's tall, dark, and handsome. Every time I dream of him, I'm intimidated. He's way out of my league. (You know what I mean, right?) The strange thing is, he's pursuing me. And in some dreams, he's my boyfriend! I used to fantasize about this type of man, but in my daydreams, I was tall, svelte, and blond. In reality, I'm a petite Korean woman, so how do I respond when he wants me just as I am—blemishes and all?

In the dream, I find it difficult to receive the attention he gives me. But the more time I spend with him, I can't resist. His eyes radiate with love.

Through these dreams, God has revealed that I can't earn his love. This is a problem, because I have difficulty receiving. It is easier to worship and love on Jesus than to sit and let him love on me.

A few months ago, I took a prayer class. One night, we spent twenty minutes adoring Jesus. Then we spent ten minutes receiving Jesus's adoration toward us. Nearly everyone shared how they enjoyed giving adoration, but they were uncomfortable receiving it. Why? Because when we receive, we're vulnerable and naked. We see our insecurity and fears, fears that say we haven't done enough to deserve His love and acceptance.

For many years, I had interpreted the Scripture to love Him with all my heart, mind, and soul as my duty. I needed to live my life where He knows I love Him. Without admitting it, I felt that once I did, I could earn His love in return. But is that how God's love works? Absolutely not!

We need to receive first in order to love.

1 John 4:10 TPT

"This is love: He loved us long before we loved him. It was his love, not ours. He proved it by sending his Son to be the pleasing sacrificial offering to take away our sins."

Perhaps you're thinking, "I'm a mess. I've fooled around with the world, and I don't deserve to receive His love." That's the enemy lying to you! God is pursuing you because He loves you.

Jesus died for your mess. Actually, He died as you — mess and all. Then He resurrected as you as well. Your former self–when you didn't know Him and fooled around with the world—has died. You're now pure and holy. That's how God sees you!

Pray.

Close your eyes and say out loud, "Jesus, show me how much You love me." Then sit still and rest in His love and acceptance.

Think.

Write Jesus a letter about what you're experiencing when you think about Him loving and adoring you. Don't hesitate to share your heart even if you're feeling afraid, ashamed, and vulnerable. He wants to know what you're thinking, feeling, and desiring from Him. Show Him your true self since this entry is only between you and Him.

Act.

Every day, spend ten minutes receiving His love. Express that you want to receive His love and envision receiving His love. I often picture myself lying on His chest while He tells me, "I love you."

Day 30: Refined Intimacy

by JennRene Owens, LMSW

Exodus 20:8-11 NLT

*[8] Remember to observe the Sabbath day by keeping it holy.
[9] You have six days each week for your ordinary work, [10] but the
seventh day is a Sabbath day of rest dedicated to the Lord your
God. On that day no one in your household may do any work.
This includes you, your sons and daughters, your male and
female servants, your livestock and any foreigners living
among you.*

There I was, finally resting into my life. I had moved cross-country from Washington, D.C. to Texas. I was living out my adventurous dreams. I sat down one evening to write my favorite author, Keri Wyatt Kent:

*I can't even begin to inform you how your ministry has brought
such calm to my life. I am so much happier. When I found your
book, I was experiencing several changes and transitions in my life.
I was just a mess. Not a literal mess, but a disorganized mess. I had
relocated from Maryland, gotten married, and started a new job.
Your book brought manna and order into my life and prepared me
for what was ahead.*

Long story short…I am MUCH BETTER!

*Now, we have Sabbath rests on a regular basis. We have more
patience with ourselves and within our souls, and it has truly
calmed me. It's allowed me to POSSESS MY SOUL. It has* also

calmed my husband and helped him to walk in greater spiritual authority and rest. This is literally a miracle. I'm serious. When we married, I knew he was a great man, I just wasn't sure I could keep up with his pace. It frightened me.

Gratefully and graciously, my life slowed down because of the wisdom offered through your books. "Rest and breathe," you said. I slowed down enough to write my book. WOW! I am almost finished. It has taken forever it seems...but God... smile. I know my book shall change lives. Thanks for passing the baton - both literally and figuratively. I am influencing lives and leaving a legacy for families. I'm fulfilling the Abrahamic Covenant: "Through you all the families of the earth shall be blessed."

I would love to say my life became better overnight.

It did not. It took practice and spending time with God to develop that rest. I call this spiritual self-care. Practicing Sabbath requires life change and discipline, but the results are amazing.

Keri wrote me back with good wishes on a steady walk with Sabbath. I remember that move in 2006 as if it were yesterday. It was frantic, yet exciting. I was very nervous. I was picking up my entire life and moving westward! My boyfriend (who's now my husband), Tim, came to D.C. on a one-way flight to help me pack. I have never been good with packing. He helped me make decisions, big and small.

We squeezed into my little car and began a thirty-six-hour trip full of laughter and nostalgia. We stayed three nights in Rochester, NY, visiting my parents. Then, we headed to Tulsa, OK to visit his parents. After one night, we were on our way to Denton, TX, where I had a new apartment waiting for me. The next two years were filled with emotional upheaval. I started a new job, and we started our relationship for real - in the same state. Although we had been courting a while, we were about to really determine whether we could stand the test of time and last in each other's presence.

Relocation, marriage, and a new job are on the psychiatrist's list of top stressful events, first compiled by Thomas Holmes and Richard Rahe in 1967[10]. In one month, I experienced all three transitions. When you're going through transitions—even happy ones—being aware of how you manage your stress level will help you immensely. Stay attuned to your mental, emotional, physical, and spiritual health. You can find the Holmes-Rahe test online to assess the types of stress in your life[11].

Sabbath can help. God actually made the day of rest one of the Ten Commandments. He took a rest after He made creation, and He expects us to do the same when we toil throughout the week.

Imagine that. God created Sabbath as a commandment! That's a decree for our good! When I reflect on the benefits I have experienced as a result of Sabbath, I can count more than I have room to mention. One benefit was simply finding a rhythm in my life. When my pace slowed down, so did my husband's. In addition, we were able to find time for play and enjoyment, and weekly enjoy each other's company. It enhanced our friendship tremendously.

God also commands us to: "Keep the Sabbath holy." But what does "keep it holy" mean? "Holy" means set apart. When you set something apart to God, He blesses it.

---

[10] Thomas Holmes & Richard Rahe, "The Social Readjustment Rating Scale," Journal of Psychosomatic Research 11, no 2 (1967):213–218.
[11] https://www.stress.org/holmes-rahe-stress-inventory/.

When you are on Sabbath:

- Be in expectation. God wants to show you how to live with good rest.

- Spend time listening for God's direction. Try talking to Him. He's a good, good Father; He will answer.

- Be present with God and family.

Life can cause you to lose touch with others, but also with yourself. Have you ever felt your head was cloudy, you couldn't think straight, felt overstimulated, or you needed some downtime but couldn't figure out how to practice it? Sabbath helps.

Ask yourself questions, self-evaluate, and get reacquainted with your true goals and objectives in life. You can stay home and just find a spot or corner to rest. I sometimes go to a cafe, leaving the comfort of home and spending time with someone else. I honor God and pursue my passion for relationship with my family in my own quirky little, peaceful way.

What's KEY during Sabbath?

Stay clear of busyness. I have done everything from scrapbooking to blogging during this Sabbath time. It cannot be stressful. If an entire day of Sabbath makes you anxious, don't allow this to impede you. One moment at a time, maybe half a day for a few weeks, will help you begin. Put the family on alert that you are beginning a new practice and set boundaries around it.

I highly recommend putting the television and phone away.

Arrange your day with a different plan—a plan for no busyness. When I relax my mind, my creativity soars. I reflect with my family, dream, and plan new activities. Sabbath offers me sanctuary. It has been fun to explore.

We all need to find time to have meaningful relationships and cherish time with our friends, children, and family. We could miss out on the best opportunities to bond, had we not learned the skill of practicing Sabbath. Instead, let's develop special rituals with those we love. The time you take to spend with your special people could be life-changing. You could share wisdom and add immensely to one another's growth and insight.

Pray.

Lord, You are the God of Rest. You lead us beside still waters. Help us know rest beside those waters and be in expectation of great resolve. When I notice my list of things to do, it's scary to take a day off. I choose to obey You in taking a Sabbath rest. I'll relax into You, spending time in prayer, reflection, and good companionship.

Think.

What can you do today to make your Sabbath plan solid?

Act.

Enjoy your Sabbath! Let it flow. Remind yourself throughout the day to notice God's presence and say hello.

Day 31: Psalmistry

by JennRene Owens, LMSW

Psalm 23:1-3 NLT

[1]The Lord is my shepherd; I have all that I need. [2]He lets me rest in green meadows; he leads me beside peaceful streams. [3]He renews my strength. He guides me along right paths, bringing honor to his name.

Many people are uncomfortable with developing margin in their life for true rest. I ask God often to help me find time for the space I need to just <u>be</u> and deal with my soul's unrest. The "art of being me" has been carefully cultivated! I take time and consideration to listen to my soul.

When I deal with high stress on the job or in life, or when I struggle with getting things done, I can forget I have a need for space. We all tend to struggle with this. We neglect family time or ignore the nudge in our spirit which says to put the phone down, be still, or sit in the bedroom with no lights on for a little while. Those sacred spaces pass right by us. We should take the opportunity to be alone.

If it's difficult to appreciate those moments, try writing a prayer or a psalm. The Psalms have inspired us for thousands of years. King David and the other psalmists poured out their fears, frustrations, adoration, and joy. Once they released what was on their minds, they were able to express faith that God would come through as He always does.

Another time in your life to write a psalm would be when you are frustrated and upset with people in your life. Maybe you have sorrow of some kind because of a relationship. God encourages us to lament, because it helps cleanse our soul from unhealthy and difficult thoughts. We all struggle with times in our lives when we are challenged with hardships. The good thing about those challenges is we can leave these God-times with a sense of relief and restored love. We feel hopeful after casting our cares on Him. We can release sorrow and frustration for not coming clean with God and be truly honest before Him.

At times, I have dealt with subtle rebellion in not desiring to do what God has shown me. I've chosen to do the opposite. This strong desire to do things my way is disobedience. Later, I have found wisdom in the Psalms as I chose to walk in peace, hope, and acquiescence. It is so much less stressful for me when I yield to Him.

During one of my Sabbath moments, I created a psalm. The intimacy I had with God was very high. It felt like a refined moment where He brought great clarity. You can write a psalm from your heart. Intentionally express trust, praise, and yes, even lament. You can complain with God. He loves when we vent! David vented often, and God called him a man after His own heart! I am learning that confession before God heals. There is safety in this type of vulnerability and exposure before God because it involves illumination and understanding.

A Psalm unto My Lord

I love the Lord because He heard my heart.
God listens to my heart like none other.
He loves me because He made me before the foundations of the earth.
Before I even existed, God ordained me to be a Healer.
I am His confidant, marked by His presence and His purpose.

When life becomes unmanageable for me,

Oh God, you bring me into a very still place and say:
"Listen."
In the hearkening of my ears Lord, You allow me to find
peace.
You wanted me to understand that
In Stillness,
In Your Rest.
In Your Purpose.
In Your Love.
In Your steadfast love - that reaches far beyond the Sun, the
Moon, and Galaxies, and Stars.
Be very near, and in Your nearness I shall have
Direction, Purpose, & Strength.
When my friends mocked me and thought I was
disillusioned they said:
"What are you doing with your life? You seem confused!"
Even the silent mocking - I still heard them, Lord.
When I wandered…seemingly purposeless and without
direction, they said:
"Where is God in that?"
Even the ones closest to me questioned my ability to
understand You, Oh God
Yet You held me close.
Speak Your love over me in waves
Waves that allow me to love You with quiet and soft music
– rocking me to sleep.
Rein me into the silence of Your love,
To love You with Sabbath simplicity, listening for what is
dear in Your heart;
Not mine.
Searching for You in the silence and resting in You, with
my whole heart.

I love You, Lord. It's because of You I have a new sense of direction.
I have a befitting and determined course.
Because of You, my heart sings praises for a new occupation
That has set me in the land of opportunity.
One without limitation, that speaks from praise and purpose;
Healing and leadership and longing.
I thank You.
Selah.

My conclusion is this:
Although there will be times in your life when you don't quite understand Your God,
Remain grateful to Him.
Remain in a state of peace and contemplation on what He said last.
Remain Hidden in that word He gave you,
And write it on your heart of remembrance
And on the walls of your living space, so it is easily read.
Trust that God has given you a vision and adhere – because the vision defines your future.
Celebrate in the quietness of God's love.
Rest Assured He will answer in the end.
The Lord loves a faithful contemplator of His word.
Selah.

I love writing to God. Writing letters to Him helps me to be more aware and alert to my prayer life. I craft my words with intention. I began this practice when I was twenty-five years old and over time, it has grown into one I find most beautiful.

I also practice a solemn process that involves practicing the Examen[12] and writing thoughts about my inner life. It brings a resolve to my soul. My friends and close family members may have noticed my resolve before I did. And yes, I attribute this to my practice of Sabbath simplicity.

Pray.

Lord, thank You for always being available through prayers and intimate writings. The fact that you desire to draw nigh even when I am complaining and frustrated - I find refuge in that. I love You. Guide me every single day and every hour. I know You've given me all the resources and talents I need to live my best life. I love knowing You'll never leave my side, and I want the world to know how good You are.

Think.

Would you like to write a note to the Option Ocean author who inspired you? Go to www.menti.com and use code 782603, or go to http://1MomentWiser.com/contact and send us an email. You can write notes to more than one of us, if you like. Words of kindness make everyone's day better.

---

[12] A technique of prayerfully reflecting upon your day to discern God's presence and direction for you. To learn more: https://www.ignatianspirituality.com/ignatian-prayer/the-examen.

Act.

Get a copy of Keri Wyatt Kent's books[13], *Breathe*, *Rest*, *Godspace*, or *Sabbath Simplicity*. Insert Sabbath time into your life and work your way up to a whole day of Sabbath each week.

---

[13] http://keriwyattkent.com/.

In Closing

"What would you tell your eighteen-year-old self?" On a hike, I pondered the question. So many things I'd say to the young, seductive, insecure Kristi Bridges. I'd probably echo what others were already telling her, but where they had concerns, I have memories. The young Kristi Bridges didn't listen to those people, but what if the advice came from me?

Lauren Daigle has a song that goes, "I believe what You say of me." After my hike, I was making a cup of chai. Lauren's song came on, and I had to put down my cup and worship. The cup includes the words of Proverbs 31:29 ESV, "You are an Amazing Woman. 'Many women have done excellently, but you surpass them all.'" It was a gift from a friend who really meant it. I am not the person Kristi Bridges thought she'd be, and I'm not the person I will be when the last page of my story is written. But it's the coolest thing—the eighteen-year-old Kristi Bridges became who I am today. She turned out confident and loving. She thinks before she speaks; therefore, she sounds more intelligent. She knows life isn't over if you haven't achieved everything by the age of twenty-five. She has a husband who encourages, respects, and loves her.

You are going to be fine. Lean on Jesus, let the Holy Spirit move you forward and love the Lord your God with every molecule and every moment.

Author Bios

Richard Staley, PhD

Day 4: Set Your Compass, Day 24: Riot or Rescue
Dr. Richard Staley discovered his calling in education. After several years as the superintendent of a school district, he returned to the classroom as a University of Missouri professor. When distance learning rose in popularity, Dr. Staley adapted. Lecturing on television and then online, he demonstrated that learning should never stop. Now retired, he is currently helping to launch an addiction recovery program in his community.

Rip Kastaris

Day 5: Picked up on a Wave, Day 6: Confluence
The son of a Greek Orthodox priest, Rip Kastaris immigrated to the United States as a young child with his family as part of his father's mission. Today, he has three children of his own. Rip graduated from Washington University in St. Louis as Valedictorian of the School of Fine Arts and has also served as an adjunct professor there. He is the first Hellenic-American to be chosen by the United States Olympic Committee (USOC) to commemorate US athletes. His award-winning Olympic works include the 2002 *Fire and Ice series*, which celebrated Olympic skiing, ice skating, and ice hockey; the *Athena* series honoring US Athletes participating in the Athens Olympiad; and the epic Olympic mural *Kyklos - Circle of Glory* in Athens Olympic Stadium. In 2018, he produced Byzantine Icons for Orthodox sanctuaries and private collections. Since 1999, he has served

as Creative Director for the Hellenic Cultural Foundation. His is based out of St. Louis, Missouri, where visitors can see his *Confluence* mural on Broadway Avenue. You can see Rip's art, as well as videos of his process at http://facebook.com/kastaris.

Cyndilu Miller

Day 7: A Pin in the Map, Day 16: Midnight Meditation
Cyndilu Miller is not just a survivor, but a leader. She knows what it's like to experience abuse and make life-altering decisions based on fear, so today she helps others find their voices, discover their gifts, and boldly live out their dreams. In one sentence, she is a globetrotting, miracle-loving, God-fearing woman who helps people see the world through new lenses. She is living life out loud through her super powers of being a Spontaneous Songstress and Speaker. She lives with her beloved husband Robin on the South Island of New Zealand. She can frequently be found racking airline miles as she travels to speak or to visit her five children and nine grandchildren in the US. You can hear her on all your favorite podcasting or social media sources. Just look for BeBOLDYou!

Sarah Soon

Day 8: Pressure v Power, Day 29: The Man of My Dreams
Sarah Soon's desire is to help people share their story, for story connects us as humans. She longs to see people discover their voice and proclaim their unique identity through their story! Sarah obtained a bachelor's in international business with a German minor before becoming a freelance writer and editor. She's edited a variety of non-fiction books, ranging from medical topics to Christian living. She's ghostwritten two memoirs for clients, as well as articles for Tulsa Lifestyle

Magazine. She blogs at WritebyGrace.com and Write2Edit.com, conducts marketing services for a wedding venue, and helps edit the blogs and newsletters of others. As a novelist and visionary, she co-created the It's About Time novel-writing course. She enjoys going on hikes and learning about different cultures. Follow her at www.Write2Edit.com to learn more about writing and editing.

Premadonna Braddick, MA

Day 11: Follow Wisdom
Premadonna Braddick is a behavioral health counselor, ordained minister, author, and actress. She's a prime example of overcoming less than desirable circumstances. In the foster care system from age two to eighteen, she spent the early years of her life dealing with depression, low self-esteem, and a poor self-image. She holds a Bachelor of Arts degree in communication with a minor in theatre arts from San Jose State University. At Oral Roberts University, she earned two Master of Arts degrees in marriage and family therapy and Christian counseling. She's a member of Delta Sigma Theta Sorority, former member of Kappa Phi Beta Honor Society and graduate from Leadership Tulsa Class 54. Mrs. Braddick received the 2018 Woman of the Year Pinnacle award from YWCA and the Mayor's Commission on the Status of Women. Recently, she was selected for the Oklahoma for Excellence award for her outstanding mentorship work with teen girls and families in the community. Her passion is the nonprofit she created, Soaring Eagles Youth and Family Services, Inc. This organization provides troubled teens with counseling, mentorship, an annual Girls' Teen Summit, health and fitness workshops, and community service. Her motto is, "When you have a set-back, don't take a step-back, because God

is already preparing your come-back!" Support Soaring Eagles at www.facebook.com/soaringeaglesyfs/.

Smiley Elmore Jr., PhD

Day 13: Recruited for the JFL
Dr. Smiley Elmore, Jr. is husband of twenty-six years to his lovely bride, Angela. He's father to their four amazing children. His mom and dad taught him the value of keeping Christ first and working extremely hard. He listened. He became an ordained minister and holds three earned academic degrees, including a PhD in Christian education. He holds the current World Record for "Most Weight Hammer-Curled in 1 Minute" at 4,000 pounds. He also holds a football record at the University of Missouri for 187 yards on eighteen carries. He was a guest star on American Gladiators and traveled the world performing feats of strength with The Power Team and The Strength Team. He and his wife recently opened Smiley Champion Fitness studio in Tulsa, OK, where they encourage children, teens, and adults to become the champions we all were created to be. Keep up with Smiley at www.facebook.com/smileychampionsfitness/.

Dr. Philip Greenaway

Day 14: God Doesn't Lie
Dr. Philip Greenaway obtained his doctorate in divinity at the International Seminary. The son of missionary parents, he has pastored four churches and led fundraising efforts for civic and humanitarian projects for the Assemblies of God World Headquarters. As the former director of development for Metro Ministries and current regional manager of Trinity Broadcasting Network, he has produced videos, created digital

materials, and managed an urban outreach. Currently, he is the pastor of Open Bible Christian Center in Massillon, Ohio, where he lives with his loving wife, Tracy. Check out his blog at http://obccmassillon.com/.

Rev. Jimmy John Sill

Day 17: The One Who Heals Me, Day 20: The One Who Sees Me
Reverend Jimmy John Sill has managed dual roles for over twenty years. With a Bachelor of Science in education from Oklahoma State University, he has served the trucking industry as an expert witness, safety strategist, mentor, trainer, and speaker. As a living witness to the healing and salvation power of our Lord Jesus Christ, he has served as a youth pastor, Royal Rangers Outpost Senior Commander, lay minister and life group leader. Today, he pastors Crosspointe Assembly of God in Sapulpa, OK. He considers himself an Eternal Life Coach helping people achieve their greatest potential by coaching, guiding, and empowering them to love God and love people. Jimmy John says, "To proclaim love is one thing, to demonstrate it is another. Being a living example of grace, mercy, and compassion is what we must do to see the world changed." Check out Crosspointe at https://www.cross pointeagsapulpa.com/.

Kim White

Day 18: Egg Escape
Kim White, founder of My Sexy Business, is an author, international speaker, collaboration specialist, influencer of influencers, and leader of mastermind groups all over the world. Her question for every entrepreneur is, "Do you own your business, or does it own you?" As a serial entrepreneur,

Kim shares her business acumen and life lessons with coaching clients, students, and members of the My Sexy Business Club. Through her *Hope to Hope* conferences, *Biz Besties* retreats, and collaboration classes, she blends memorable experiences with opportunities for skill development, strategic planning, and high-quality networking. Learn from her at www.facebook.com/princesskimwhite.

Debra Trappen

Day 21: Embracing Self-Love

Debra Trappen's book, *Fire Up! Taking Your Life and Business to 11*, began a movement. A motivational speaker, trainer, podcaster, and author, she founded her company to serve growth-minded leaders. She concentrates on engaging, elevating, and empowering women. She can help you define, design, and intentionally live your signature life out loud, serve your communities, and become the change you wish to see - all with a fiery focus, confidence, and purpose. When she is not idea-storming her next adventure or writing, interviewing, or recording in her Fire Up studio, you will find her enjoying quiet time devouring books and podcasts, walking her pups, watching Sci-Fi flicks, or wine tasting with her hubby across the globe for her passion project, WomenOnWine. Visit Debra at https://debratrappen.com.

JennRene Owens, LMSW

Day 30: Refined Intimacy, Day 31: Psalmistry

With a burden for those who silently endure challenges, Jennifer Owens strives to help people find beauty in their own vulnerability. She's the author of *Red Sea Situations: Finding Courage in the Deep Seas of Life* and the creator of the self-care course, *The Rhythm Conscious Life*. Jennifer also helps writers craft their life stories and walk in greater purpose and intention. With a master's degree from the Howard University School of Social Work, she has served the public for over twenty years as a social worker, certified mental health therapist, resident chaplain, speaker, and leadership coach. Winner of the 2003 Diversity Achievers Award for the Central New York YWCA leaders, she has been a host, co-creator, and honored guest at several conferences, including *A Rose in Bloom; Diamonds: Understanding the Value of Being God's True Jewel*, and *Women Who Are Able to Produce*. Her passion for interviewing, creating documentaries and leading group discussions opened the door for her to teach as an adjunct professor in New York and participate in youth dialogue sessions in South Africa. Read Jennifer's blog at https://jennrene.com.

Kristi Bridges

Day 1: Who are you? Ask the I AM, Day 2: Kryptonite, Day 3: Zone of Genius, Day 9: Your Real Name, Day 10: PICK Your Life, Day 12: Difficult People, Day 15: Tough Stuff, Day 19: Boundaries, Day 22: Competitive, Day 23: Headwinds v Tailwinds, Day 25: Truth Pact Part 1, Day 26: Truth Pact Part 2, Day 27: Lead

Kristi Bridges is the author of *Yes, Please! With Sprinkles*, the *Wisdom – Better than Wishing* book and journal, *Fred O and Pumpy* and over 300 poems and songs. She hosts the 1 Moment Wiser daily devotional on YouTube, Twitter, and Facebook, as well as the *1 Moment Wiser* podcast. "You've seen that person walking nose-to-device, heading for a pole? I like preventing bloody noses," Kristi says. It's her mission to help people live wisely, avoid regret and connect with their

Creator. We change the world when we share what God has taught us, so Kristi created the *Share Your Wisdom Wisely Devotional Book Writing Experience*. As a coach with Where We Belong Family Stories, she helps people preserve generations of memories. Stories have power, so she and fellow author Sarah Soon created the *It's About Time* novel-writing workshop series. Find Kristi on your favorite social media or podcasting site, or visit her website, http://1MomentWiser.com. Her husband of twenty-two years, Richard Staley, makes sure she laughs every day. Richard is the son of Dr. Staley, one of our authors.

CPSIA information can be obtained
at www.ICGtesting.com
Printed in the USA
FFHW021717180519
52512750-57944FF